I love this book! It's both hugely informat  three-step model to support their own we
  – Brendan O'Sullivan Lic AC, MBAcC

Whilst modern medicine focuses on medication rather than looking at the root cause, the link that this book makes between diet and mental health makes complete sense.
  – Jayne Oliver RN, NMP

Joanne Mordue explains clearly and succinctly how to manage diet, lifestyle and the nervous system in order to achieve a more balanced, harmonious relationship between them. This book highlights the connections between the physical, cognitive and emotional parts of ourselves and the importance of attending to each of these in order to achieve good health. It's user friendly with lots of helpful tasks, links, recipes and tips, and Joanne is honest about the difficulties many of us have in making changes. Her approach is supportive and encouraging and I found her openness about her own journey made me want to read on and start making small changes immediately.
  – Sara Ward BSc (Hons) Psychology, BSc (Hons) Ayurvedic MA

Joanne Mordue's excellent nutritional support has helped me through irritable bowel syndrome and the menopause and is still helping me with my depression.
  – Beryl, client

Joanne Mordue is a gem! My original consultation was after a diagnosis of IBS. I didn't mention my problems with depression at first because I assumed nutritional therapy wouldn't help. But after following the three-point plan for a few months, I felt so much better both mentally and physically.
  – Lisa, client

After discovering I was vitamin deficient, I followed Joanne's recommendations to the letter and the improvement in my mental health has been life changing.
  – Alison, client

My depression got much better after following Joanne Mordue's nutrition advice.

– Joanne, client

I've had low-level depression for as long as I can remember. Nothing seemed to help. A friend recommended I see Joanne Mordue. I've been following the three-point plan for a couple of years now and I estimate that I feel about 70 per cent better than before. Results have been slow but steady.

– Becky, client

I felt like I was going crazy because every blood test the doctors and specialists recommended came back normal. I didn't know vitamin deficiencies could cause mental health problems. My mental health is now massively better and I feel physically better as well. I'll never go back to my old way of eating.

– Laura, client

I highly recommend Joanne Mordue's book. I found it outstanding. Joanne's nutrition recommendations helped me control my acid reflux naturally with diet and nutrition supplements. In this book are the keys to a healthy gut, which is essential to good health, both physically and mentally.

– Linda, client

My daughter was struggling to attend school because of ADHD and high anxiety; her stress and unhappiness was upsetting for all the family. I never considered food allergies could contribute to her problems, but after cutting out the allergic foods my daughter is now much calmer. She no longer needs medication, she sleeps well and her school attendance is much improved

– Sarah, a relieved parent

When I first heard Joanne Mordue explaining the physical cause behind some people's mental illness I was intrigued. I had some tests which helped me understand why I felt the way I did. I now take supplements every day, follow Joanne's diet advice and I feel much better.

– Meriel, client

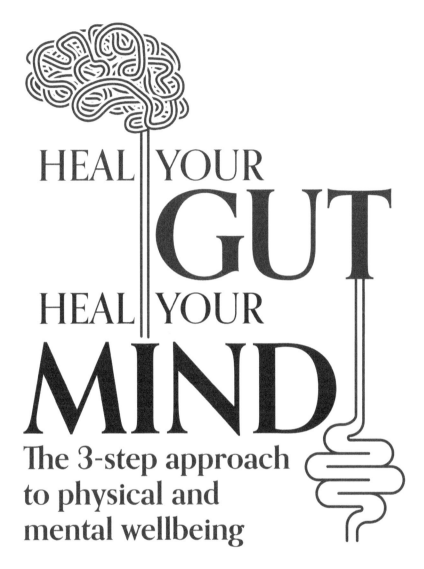

HEAL YOUR GUT

HEAL YOUR MIND

The 3-step approach to physical and mental wellbeing

JOANNE MORDUE

FOREWORD BY PATRICK HOLFORD

Heal Your Gut, Heal Your Mind

ISBN 978-1-915483-10-2 (paperback)
ISBN 978-1-915483-11-9 (ebook)

Published in 2025 by Right Book Press
Printed in the UK

This book is dedicated to God, for blessing me with the grace to create this book.

And to Guy Marshall – my life partner, my love, my greatest supporter.

Disclaimer

I recommend consulting your doctor about the symptoms you're experiencing and any dietary changes you're planning to make, as well as any supplements you want to take. Some nutritional supplements may interact with other medications, so always check with your GP first. The content of this book should not be considered a substitute for professional medical advice and I am not a qualified medical practitioner.

My case studies provide examples of the results of my three-point plan approach but should not be regarded as concrete evidence of treatment effectiveness.

To be clear, I'm not the first person to make the recommendations laid out in this book. In doing so, I'm standing on the shoulders of giants in the orthomolecular field of medicine. However, I believe, perhaps for the first time, my book puts the pieces of the jigsaw together and offers a simple, easy-to-follow plan for recovery from gut and brain symptoms.

I'm not entirely comfortable with the term 'mental illness' and will be explaining why. But for the purpose of this book and descriptive uses only, I will be using the term. No disrespect is intended.

All of the recommendations I make in this book are genuine and based on my personal experience. I am not financially benefiting from any of them.

Contents

Foreword

There is a strange and obvious thing that is usually ignored, and which this book sets straight. The mind is connected to the brain, which is part of the body, which is literally made from the food that is digested and absorbed through the gut. In other words, what you eat and what goes on in your gut directly affects how you think and feel.

In this book you'll find a number of rich avenues to explore if you are suffering from either mental health issues or gut issues, or both. Through the author's own journey she has discovered keystones for not only mental and gut health but all health. She pieces together the jigsaw and shows you how to climb the ladder towards robust gut and mental health. I call it the soil–food–gut–brain superhighway. The soil, like us, has a microbiome, which should be a rich field of organisms, our allies in being healthy. In the soil it makes healthy plants, which we then eat. But this understanding is not well acknowledged and as a consequence, the standard path of modern living, diet and lifestyle too often leads to mental health problems that cannot be solved by pharmaceuticals because a lack of drugs was never part of the cause.

By looking from the gut towards the brain, Joanne gives you tremendous insight and avenues to explore and resolve, to allow your mind and body to return to good health. Enjoy the journey of discovery and recovery.

Patrick Holford, founder of the Institute for Optimum Nutrition, Food for the Brain Foundation (foodforthebrain.org) and author of *Upgrade Your Brain* (2024).

Introduction

My story

Everyone has their own back story – their own personal set of circumstances that led to digestive and/or mental health problems. This is mine...

I first started displaying digestive and mental health symptoms as a teenager, but I believe the cause of my illness was cumulative and started many years before. I was breastfed as a baby, which gave me a great start in life. It contributed towards me having healthy gut bacteria, and as a child, my digestion was robust. But unfortunately, I was a very anxious child, and stress negatively affects our digestive system in many ways.

My anxiety worsened when I moved to a new school. At 13 years old, leaving my friends and adapting to a new school environment felt pretty traumatic. Chronic, prolonged stress and unhappiness culminated in me developing a panic disorder. I had daily panic attacks that became so severe I could no longer attend school and had to be home-schooled.

As I previously mentioned, stress is bad for digestion – and panic attacks provoke a severe stress response in the body. So, as a stressed and unhappy teenager, my gut health was most certainly compromised. However, I still wasn't displaying any gut symptoms.

Around this time, I developed acne and my doctor prescribed antibiotics that I took constantly for many years. They helped to improve the appearance of my skin – but at a high price. I only wish I'd had the knowledge I have now. If I'd been aware of the damage long-term antibiotic use was doing to my gut, I would never have taken them. Instead, I'd have lovingly embraced my spotty face!

Antibiotics kill bacteria. Full stop. They don't differentiate between beneficial bacteria and bad bacteria and only kill the bad – they kill both (Bradley 2023). An average course of antibiotics only lasts a week or two, and our gut bacteria can just about maintain a healthy balance during this time. But my GP prescribed them for several years, so my poor gut bacteria didn't stand a chance.

My anxiety lessened upon leaving school but then, at around the age of 19, I started taking the contraceptive pill. The pill can raise copper levels (Crews et al 1980), which may trigger anxiety and panic for some people. My panic attacks returned with a vengeance, then unpleasant digestive symptoms developed and quickly became severe, along with other issues such as recurrent yeast infections and fatigue.

Around this time, I had a hospital appointment with a dermatologist. He wanted to prescribe a powerful drug called isotretinoin (more commonly known to the layperson by its brand name, Roaccutane). I'd taken it a couple of years previously and it had cleared up my acne, but only temporarily. The list of its side effects is extensive and they can be severe (according to the UK government, these can include depression, anxiety and psychotic symptoms – see MHRA 2020). I tried to discuss my concerns about the effect of such a powerful drug on my digestive system and my overall health, but he rudely pooh-poohed everything I said and denied there was any link between my declining health and my long-term use of prescription drugs. But I trusted my gut instinct and began to do my own research, and realised that the deterioration in my health was largely due to my damaged gut flora and fauna. I said no to the isotretinoin and stopped the antibiotics and the contraceptive pill, and instead took a more natural and gentle approach to my health.

I read a wonderful book which sparked my passion for nutrition called *Erica White's Beat Candida Cookbook* (2014). *Candida albicans* is a pathogenic yeast that lives harmlessly in the human gut, but when gut bacteria get out of balance (as in the case of long-term antibiotic use), *Candida* can proliferate out of control, which causes many nasty symptoms. Erica White is a nutritional therapist who studied with my nutritional guru Patrick Holford (who wrote the Foreword to this book). He takes a holistic view of illness – that is to say, he takes into account the body as a whole and treats the cause rather than the symptoms of an illness.

I followed Erica's dietary recommendations, which were basically to cut out all sugars, yeasts and processed foods and take supplements that would kill the *Candida* and support my body to heal and return to full health. I followed her recommendations religiously, and can honestly say the improvements in my health were miraculous. My digestion returned to normal, my acne vanished, and my panic attacks decreased.

The final step of my healing journey came years later when I read several books about orthomolecular medicine, which is the treatment of disease using nutrients such as vitamins and minerals. This made perfect sense to me – after all, vitamins and minerals are *essential*, and even mild deficiencies may cause the workings of the body to malfunction. So, I paid privately for blood tests to discover whether I had any vitamin and mineral deficiencies. They showed I had elevated copper levels, which can be a cause of mental illness (Chen et al 2023). The tests also showed I was chronically deficient in B6 and zinc, and a urine test showed high levels of kryptopyrroles. These rob the body of B6 and zinc and cause a recognised condition called pyrrole disorder (Cherney 2023). I researched copper overload and pyrrole disorder so that I could better understand my diagnosis, and discovered I had practically every symptom: mental health problems triggered during puberty, a family history of mental illness, food intolerances, crowded upper front teeth, insomnia, skin sensitivity, morning nausea and many more classic symptoms too numerous to list here. I was delighted to have a diagnosis and a reason for my panic disorder, but I also felt bitterly disappointed that none of the doctors or psychotherapists I had consulted over the years had suggested there could be a biological cause of my mental health problems.

I was led to believe it was 'all in my mind' and the medical profession had offered me only tranquillisers and counselling, neither of which could cure the root cause of my mental health issues. Sadly, this is all too common. Pharmaceutical drugs have their place and there have been occasions when I've had a stinker of a panic attack when I was grateful for diazepam. Talking therapy also has its place. After my diagnosis and treatment of pyrrole disorder and copper overload, cognitive behavioural therapy was helpful in breaking the cycle of negative thoughts and fears I had about panic attacks. But it was frankly a waste of time having counselling before I'd discovered and treated the root cause of my panic disorder: elevated copper, pyrrole disorder and compromised gut health.

My personal healing journey inspired my passion for nutrition and prompted me to study to become a nutritional therapist. I absolutely love my work. Helping my clients to help themselves and witnessing their return to health has been wonderfully rewarding and joyous. But I didn't start my nutrition career intending to specialise in digestive and mental health problems. It happened inadvertently because they're both so prevalent – and of course my personal experience helped me to understand my clients' problems. Over the years, I developed a three-point approach to healing: diet changes, lifestyle changes and nutritional supplements, which I call my three-point plan. This has become a way of life for me. Clean eating, taking vitamin and mineral supplements, daily breathing exercises, cold showers, meditation and fortnightly acupuncture are all essential for me to maintain optimum health.

You can see from my story that holistic healing can take time and effort. In a society where we're conditioned to take a pill as a 'quick fix' to feel better, it can be tough to find the motivation to take responsibility for your own health. I'm hopeful that your recovery will be much quicker than mine because the information in this book will guide you. I'm confident you can be well again, so trust the process and approach it as a gentle cross-country jog and not a 100-metre sprint. Good luck – you've got this.

Let's begin...

The information in this book is designed to help you take back control of your health and find freedom from all of your unpleasant symptoms. I know from my own and my clients' experience that you can be symptom free: you can feel well again. Symptoms vary from person to person and for this reason not everything I discuss will apply to you. So, I recommend reading the book with a marker pen to highlight the parts that apply to you so you can easily refer back to them.

I qualified as a nutritional therapist 15 years ago and in that time, I've discovered that most conditions can be helped by sound nutrition. Over the years I've given consultations to clients for a variety of complaints, including menopausal symptoms, high cholesterol, obesity and irritable bowel syndrome. Issues related to digestion are extremely widespread, and as more and more clients came to me for help with their digestive problems, I became something of a digestion enthusiast!

A high percentage of my clients with digestive troubles also had mental health problems, usually anxiety and/or depression. In my practice I would estimate that around 90 per cent of the people who consulted me about their digestive health were also suffering from mental health symptoms. It was interesting to observe that as my clients' digestion improved, so too did their mental health – and usually at a similar rate and to a similar extent. This implied to me that they were intimately connected, and so began my fascination with the gut–brain connection. Over time, I developed my three-pronged approach to treating my clients' digestive and mental health. I call this my three-point plan.

» **Point 1: Dietary changes.** One of the best ways to achieve equilibrium in both body and mind is to eat a healthy diet full of nutrient-dense foods while removing nutritionally deficient ones. Eating the wrong foods for you can trigger both digestive and emotional symptoms.

» **Point 2: Lifestyle changes**. Lifestyle factors such as stress, unhappiness, loneliness and a lack of self-care can also cause digestive and emotional troubles. Simple lifestyle changes such as relaxation techniques, positive thinking, group activities and nurturing oneself can have huge health benefits.

» **Point 3: Nutritional supplements**. Supplements are just what their name suggests – they supplement a healthy diet by aiding digestion, healing the gut and correcting deficiencies. Anyone with digestive troubles or high stress levels is unlikely to be absorbing all of the vitamins and minerals from their food. Even mild vitamin and mineral deficiencies can have a profoundly negative effect on physical and mental health, so I believe supplements are an essential part of recovery.

This approach to health could be called lifestyle or functional medicine. It's a holistic method that takes a personal approach to healing and deals with the cause and prevention of disease rather than taking a pill to suppress the symptoms. Treating my clients as a whole and recognising that everything in the body is intimately connected is essential to their recovery. It's a bit like piecing together a jigsaw puzzle. For true healing to occur, we must take into account emotional, physical and environmental factors. All too often the focus is on suppressing the symptoms of disease with prescription medication rather than treating the cause of disease. This often leads to more and more pills being prescribed to suppress the side effects of the initial medication!

I believe that mental healthcare is failing some people in the Western world. Antidepressants, tranquillisers and talking therapy all have a role to play but no one seems to be asking the question, why are mental health problems dramatically increasing year on year? Why are more and more people being prescribed antidepressants? What has changed to cause mental health issues, digestive issues and many other major diseases to increase at such a frightening rate? Well, I think my three-point plan provides some big clues. Over the past 75 years, our diet has changed faster than at any other point in our evolution, as has our lifestyle. As a result, many people are nutritionally deficient without even realising it. An analysis in *The Lancet* found that diet is involved in one in five deaths (GBD 2017 Diet Collaborators 2019). No amount of prescription medicine can fix this alarming healthcare crisis. I passionately believe that there should be more research into diet and environmental factors as a way to prevent illness.

This book aims to help you understand what's going on in your body to cause your symptoms and gives you an action plan to help you return to full health. As you follow my three-point plan and your digestion, mental health and vitamin status improve, you may notice your overall health improving too. You should have more energy, more clarity of mind, you'll sleep better, aches and pains will ease, the condition of your skin should improve and many other things that are not obviously related will all improve. This is because good health really does start and end in the gut. I hope you find this book helpful and inspiring and I wish you well on your road to recovery.

Part 1

Freedom from gut and brain symptoms

Chapter 1

Food, mood and poop journal

A food, mood and poop journal is a tool for tracking what you eat, your emotional state and your digestive symptoms. This information is invaluable in regaining control of your health. Keeping a journal has many benefits: it's a brilliant way to see the link between the foods we eat and the way we feel, it shows you where you need to make changes, it keeps you accountable and it helps you recognise the connection between your digestive and mental health. The bottom line is that keeping a food, mood and poop journal is a fantastic tool.

The reason I've put this chapter at the beginning of the book is to give you the opportunity to start your journal today. So, by the time you've finished this book, you'll be ready to start implementing my three-point plan and recording your progress. I'd like you to record at least a fortnight's worth of your current diet so you can compare how you feel now with how you feel when you're following my three-point plan. Try to make this fortnight as typical as possible to give the most accurate picture.

Another important reason to start this now is that you can show your GP the changes you're making. It will be helpful for them to assess whether your diet and health have improved. When making dietary changes, there's always the concern that excluding certain food groups will make you vitamin deficient. If you eat the full range of foods I recommend in this book, I'm confident your diet will be more nutrient dense than a typical Western diet.

Keep your food, mood and poop journal with you all day and write down everything immediately – don't rely on your memory at the end of the day.

How to fill out the food, mood and poop journal

Food and drink

In this column, write down exactly what you ate. For example, if you ate pie and chips, don't forget to mention the gravy you poured over them. Also, in this column, note down when you take your supplements. If you're taking the same ones every day, there's no need to write each of them down every single day. Just note the time and mention if you add any new supplements or stop taking any.

Quantity

When describing the quantity of your main meal, put it all on your plate, then clench your fist and estimate how many fists are on your plate. Bear in mind that your stomach is roughly the same size as your clenched fist, so to eat any more than this in one sitting will overload your stomach and impair digestion. You might prefer to measure in another way, and that's OK too.

Activity

In this column, write down what you were doing while eating or drinking. For example, 'nothing' or 'sitting at my laptop working'. My advice is to always sit down and eat your food in a mindful fashion. Chew thoroughly and take your time.

Example of a food, mood and poop journal

EXAMPLE FOOD AND MOOD DIARY

TIME	FOOD & DRINK - INC SUPPLEMENTS	QUANTITY	ACTIVITY WHILE EATING	HOW YOU FEEL EMOTIONALLY?	HOW DO YOU FEEL PHYSICALLY?	BOWEL MOVEMENTS	STRESS MANAGEMENT
Midnight - 2 am							
2am - 4am							
4am - 6am					WIDE AWAKE		
6am - 8am	TEA, TOAST & JAM	1 CUP / 2 SLICES	AT HOME WATCHING TV	FEELING LOW	TIRED		
8am - 10am					TUMMY ACHE		
10am - 12 Noon						DIARRHOEA	
12 Noon - 2pm							YOGA CLASS
2pm - 4pm	COFFEE & CAKE	1 CUP / 1 SLICE	YOGA STUDIO, CHATTING	UPLIFTED	ENERGISED		
4pm - 6pm						DIARRHOEA	
6pm - 8pm	CHICKEN PIE, CHIPS AND BEANS	3 FISTS	AT HOME CHATTING	FEELING LOW	TIRED		
8pm - 10pm	CUP OF TEA						
10pm - Midnight					EXHAUSTED BUT CAN'T SLEEP		

ON A SCORE OF 1 TO 10, HOW HAVE YOU FELT PHYSICALLY? 5

HOW HAVE YOU FELT EMOTIONALLY? 5

ADDITIONAL NOTES - IBS Seems worse when I don't sleep well.

Blank Food and Mood Diary

TIME	FOOD & DRINK - INC SUPPLEMENTS	QUANTITY	ACTIVITY WHILE EATING	HOW DO YOU FEEL EMOTIONALLY?	HOW DO YOU FEEL PHYSICALLY?	BOWEL MOVEMENTS	STRESS MANAGEMENT
Midnight - 2 am							
2am - 4am							
4am - 6am							
6am - 8am							
8am - 10am							
10am - 12 Noon							
12 Noon - 2pm							
2pm - 4pm							
4pm - 6pm							
6pm - 8pm							
8pm - 10pm							
10pm - Midnight							

ON A SCORE OF 1 TO 10, HOW HAVE YOU FELT PHYSICALLY?

HOW HAVE YOU FELT EMOTIONALLY?

Printable copies of the food, mood and poop journal are available to download at www.joannemordue.com

Mood

Note how you feel emotionally while eating and drinking and, if you notice a change in your emotions at any other time of day, note this down also.

How you feel physically

In this column, record all your physical symptoms while you're eating and throughout the rest of the day – for example, stomach cramps, windy, tired, headache.

Bowel movements

Please note down every time you go to the toilet, even if you're so constipated you can't manage a bowel movement. Please give a brief description — for example, small pellets with mucus, moderate diarrhoea or severe diarrhoea. Alternatively, you could use the Bristol Stool Chart (see References and resources) and just write down the corresponding number.

Stress management

Include at least one period of relaxation every day. I will be giving you ideas and suggestions in the chapter about lifestyle changes. It can sometimes take a little bit of time to get used to incorporating 'you time' into your daily routine. Your journal will help you stay accountable. This is an integral part of your stress management and an essential part of your recovery. So, find something you enjoy and take pleasure in. For example, a walk, a bath, reading, yoga, meditation, singing, colouring in – anything that brings down your stress levels.

At the end of each day, rate how you've felt overall, mentally and physically – 0 being not good at all and 10 being great. For example, if you've felt really depressed, you'd probably give a low score – maybe a 2. If you've had a good day free from symptoms, you might feel like giving yourself a high score, say a 9.

Additional notes

At the end of the day, include anything else you think is important. For example, if you exercised, note what you did and how it made you feel. If you've excluded any food groups, you should make a note of this. And likewise, when you reintroduce foods, make a note. You could also note any test results. Another thing to note is your sleep. Many people find a lack of sleep can exacerbate their symptoms. I can't stress enough how important a food, mood and poop journal is on your road to recovery, so do your best to make the time and effort needed. It's all an investment in your health.

Take action

» Make photocopies of the food, mood and poop journal and put them in a folder.
» Keep a blank one with you all day so that you can fill it in on the go.
» Keep your food, mood and poop journal for at least a fortnight before starting my three-point plan.

Working with your doctor

The information recorded in your journal will be helpful to your doctor so take it along with you to appointments. I recommend recording your doctor's visits in your food, mood and poop journal. Note down your conversations and how you feel about your visits. Often, it's after a doctor's appointment when you remember things – so make sure you record everything, then you can discuss them on your next visit.

If your doctor refers you to a gastroenterologist for exploratory procedures or recommends any blood tests, I recommend you always ask for a printout of your test results because it's good to know precisely what your results are. Sometimes results might only just be in the normal range, and it's helpful to know if you're borderline. Being told your results are 'normal' might lull you into a false sense of security when, in fact, you should be keeping a close eye on things and probably get retested within six months. Put any results in your food, mood and poop journal because they're all a part of your healing journey.

A BBC news article published in 2018 highlighted the limited amount of training in diet and nutrition given to medical students (Dillon 2018). This small amount of time doesn't support the growing body of evidence that food and nutrition are core to health. Hopefully, this will change because many modern diseases can be traced back to a poor diet.

There's a chance that your symptoms aren't connected to the foods you eat, but a clean diet should be the cornerstone of any healing programme. If you've already started your food journal before you visit your doctor, hopefully you'll be able to point out some correlations between what you eat and your symptoms. So, try to find a doctor who's interested in and supportive of any dietary changes you'd like to make.

Chapter 2

The gut microbiome

The gut microbiome is a fancy name for the bacteria that live in your digestive tract. Everyone's gut has a mixture of both 'good' and 'bad' bacteria. In a healthy gut, the good bacteria outnumber the bad guys and keep them in check. Digestive troubles start when this delicate balance of microbes is upset, and the bad bacteria start to outnumber the good. This is why people take probiotics, because they promote and replenish the good stuff. Probiotic drinks and supplements have become very popular, so you may have heard of them.

Did you know that the health of your gut microbiome affects most of your bodily functions? For example, your gut plays an essential part in detoxification. If your body's detox system isn't working efficiently then you'll feel sluggish, tired and headachey. Your gut microbiome also influences your immune system because 70 per cent of the cells that make up your immune system are housed in your gut, so a compromised gut microbiome may lead to recurrent colds and infections. The gut microbiome also plays an important role in mental health. One example of this is that serotonin, the happiness neurotransmitter, is produced in the gut (Cresci & Bawden 2015).

Another function of the gut microbiome is to make vitamins and minerals, but an imbalance of bacteria hinders this production, contributing to vitamin and mineral deficiency. Vitamins and minerals play a part in all bodily functions and so, as you become more and more depleted, you can become trapped in a downward spiral of poor mental and physical health.

So, as you can see, if your gut microbiome is out of kilter, there's a good chance you'll feel under the weather. A healthy gut really is the cornerstone of good health. There's more and more evidence showing that many modern-day diseases begin in the gut (Lyon 2018). The good news is that this means good health also starts in the gut – and this book will show you how.

Role and functions of the gut microbiome

Let's have a look at the role and functions of the gut microbiome. It:

» makes vitamins
» aids digestion of food
» aids absorption of nutrients
» makes neurotransmitters, including serotonin
» maintains pH balance in the gut
» maintains the integrity of the gut lining
» neutralises toxic substances such as alcohol
» boosts immunity
» fights infections
» repairs the digestive tract
» reduces allergic response to food
» reduces inflammation
» aids detoxification.

You can see from the list above how important the gut microbiome is. As Hippocrates, the ancient Greek physician, said: 'Disease begins in the gut.' But don't despair if you suspect your gut microbiome is out of whack because you can positively alter your gut microbes through a few simple diet and lifestyle changes.

The destruction of the gut microbiome

So, how does the gut microbiome get out of balance? The question in today's modern world is: how can it not? Medications such as the contraceptive pill and antibiotics, processed foods, unfiltered drinking water, alcohol, stress, smoking, lack of sleep, environmental pollutants (Singh et al 2022), chemicals, perfumes, cleaning products, pesticides, depression, anxiety, trauma and even caesarean birth may all contribute towards the destruction of the gut microbiome.

We're living in unprecedented times. No other generation in history has ingested this amount of chemicals and unnatural foods and lived at our fast, disconnected pace of life. These changes have occurred quickly, so our brain and gut defences haven't had time to evolve against the assault. Our ancestors had a much greater assortment of healthy gut bacteria than we do today. Unfortunately, each generation's gut bacteria is getting less and less diverse (Van der Vossen et al 2023).

Gut dysbiosis

Gut dysbiosis is the technical name for an imbalanced gut microbiome. When your gut doesn't have enough good bacteria to keep things in check, it allows bad bacteria to flourish and take hold. This is gut dysbiosis and it's reaching pandemic proportions (Hrncir 2022). When I explain gut dysbiosis to my clients, I compare the gut to a garden. A healthy gut microbiome is like a garden full of beautiful flowers and the things we ingest either fertilise our garden or destroy it. When dysbiosis occurs, the flowers start to die and the weeds take over.

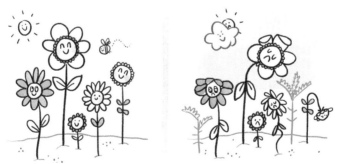

Interesting titbit
Did you know that gut dysbiosis can be caused by dysbiosis in the mouth? So take care of your oral hygiene.

Here's a quick question for you. Take a look at the drawings of the fish below and decide how you can best help the poorly one. Should you give the poorly fish medicine or should you clean its environment? Western medicine is often disease orientated rather than health orientated, so a GP might advise you to medicate the fish to treat the symptoms of its disease. On the other hand, lifestyle medicine would advise you to clean up the fish's internal and external environment in order to treat the cause of disease. Germs and disease are less likely to take hold in a healthy terrain. This is why a happy gut microbiome is so important.

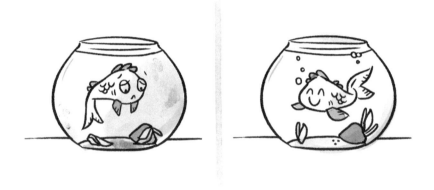

I like to show these fish drawings to my clients to help them understand that taking antacids, painkillers and other medications isn't usually treating the root cause of their poor health. What you need to do is clean up your environment by changing your diet and making a few small lifestyle changes. I understand that this can feel like hard work and popping a pill to mask your symptoms seems so much easier, but taking responsibility for your own health every day is the only way to achieve blooming health and longevity. Recent studies into epigenetics are showing that the cause of most disease is not solely down to your genes. It is, in fact, the effect your environment is having on your genes (Hunter 2005). This is great news because much of your environment (the foods you eat, the chemicals you expose yourself to) is within your control!

Do you have gut dysbiosis?

Look at each of the items below and select 0 if it's not a problem for you at all and 10 if it's a severe or regular symptom.

Constipation	0	1	2	3	4	5	6	7	8	9	10
Mucus in your stools	0	1	2	3	4	5	6	7	8	9	10
Diarrhoea	0	1	2	3	4	5	6	7	8	9	10
The feeling of incomplete bowel movements	0	1	2	3	4	5	6	7	8	9	10
Food sensitivities /intolerances	0	1	2	3	4	5	6	7	8	9	10
Poor appetite	0	1	2	3	4	5	6	7	8	9	10
Increased appetite	0	1	2	3	4	5	6	7	8	9	10
Gas and bloating	0	1	2	3	4	5	6	7	8	9	10
Indigestion	0	1	2	3	4	5	6	7	8	9	10
Abdominal pain	0	1	2	3	4	5	6	7	8	9	10
Nausea	0	1	2	3	4	5	6	7	8	9	10
Haemorrhoids	0	1	2	3	4	5	6	7	8	9	10
Stomach pain that's worse after eating and better after pooping	0	1	2	3	4	5	6	7	8	9	10
Stomach cramps	0	1	2	3	4	5	6	7	8	9	10
Reduced sex drive	0	1	2	3	4	5	6	7	8	9	10
Pain during sex	0	1	2	3	4	5	6	7	8	9	10
Recurrent vaginal thrush	0	1	2	3	4	5	6	7	8	9	10
Incontinence	0	1	2	3	4	5	6	7	8	9	10
Anxiety	0	1	2	3	4	5	6	7	8	9	10
Depression	0	1	2	3	4	5	6	7	8	9	10
Insomnia	0	1	2	3	4	5	6	7	8	9	10
Low energy and fatigue	0	1	2	3	4	5	6	7	8	9	10
Headaches/migraines	0	1	2	3	4	5	6	7	8	9	10
Skin problems such as acne or rashes	0	1	2	3	4	5	6	7	8	9	10
Storing fat around your abdomen	0	1	2	3	4	5	6	7	8	9	10
Frequent illness/infection	0	1	2	3	4	5	6	7	8	9	10
Food cravings	0	1	2	3	4	5	6	7	8	9	10

If five or more of these symptoms are a persistent problem for you, you may have gut dysbiosis. I recommend you fill out this questionnaire every few weeks while following my three-point plan, so that you can monitor your progress.

Red flags

So, now you know what gut dysbiosis is and what might be triggering it. But it's equally important to be clear about what gut dysbiosis is not, so that you don't miss any warning signs of a more serious disease such as bowel cancer. Early diagnosis is key in the treatment of bowel cancer, so it's important not to miss any obvious symptoms (also known as red flags) such as:

» weight loss
» fever
» blood in your poop
» anaemia
» tummy ache and pain during the night
» a lump in your tummy.

Please don't panic if you have any of these symptoms. They can all be related to gut dysbiosis, but it's important to discuss them with your GP so that they can decide whether to refer you for further tests. My responsibility as a nutritionist is to be aware of what my clients are presenting with and to make sure they get the right treatment.

The gut microbiome and brain health

Did you know that your gut and brain are connected? They're talking to each other all the time! The gut–brain axis is a communication network that allows the brain to influence gut activity, and the gut to influence mood and mental health (Appleton 2018). We don't know whether the gut starts the conversation or whether it's the brain, but we do know it's bidirectional. If I had to guess, I would say that it's the gut that starts the conversation, which is why mental wellbeing depends on a healthy digestive system. What's fascinating is that the type of communication between the gut and brain varies in each person – sometimes massively – and this is due to the gut health of the individual. And what determines gut health? It's our microbiome! So people with gut dysbiosis who have large amounts of bad bacteria in their gut are more likely to suffer from poor mental health (Sasso et al 2023).

The vagus nerve

This is part of the gut–brain axis. One of the ways in which the gut communicates with the brain is when the gut microbes stimulate the vagus nerve. *Vagus* is Latin for 'wandering', which describes exactly what the vagus nerve does. It wanders all over the body, connecting everything, including the gut, to the brain. It's like a communication superhighway, and it reports back to the brain exactly what's going on in the body.

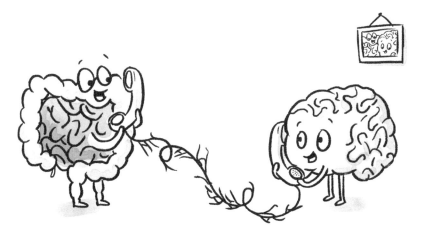

The health of the gut microbiome affects the health of the vagus nerve, which profoundly influences our mood, behaviour and overall mental health (Han et al 2022). One of the functions of the vagal feedback signals is to protect you. You know when you get a 'gut feeling' about something? Well, that comes from your vagus nerve. But poor digestive health can cause inflammation, which hinders these protective vagus signals. So, what can you do to strengthen the vagus nerve and improve the communication between your gut and your brain? I think the two most important things you can do are to rebalance the gut microbiome and reduce your stress levels.

Chapter 3

Brain symptoms

In this section, I will explore the connection between mental health, gut health and vitamin deficiencies. Research has shown that more than 50 per cent of people with irritable bowel syndrome have also been diagnosed with a mental health issue such as anxiety or depression (Kawoos et al 2017). If you have mental health and digestive problems, you will most likely be intuitively aware of a link between the two.

Think of your gut as your second brain! The digestive system contains a multitude of neurons called the enteric nervous system and it has often been called the 'second brain' because it 'feels', which directly affects our first brain (Mayer 2011). It may not be able to compose music or solve equations but the second brain influences our state of mind because our emotions are influenced by the nerves in the gut. Think of the last time you experienced butterflies in your tummy. It probably affected your emotions more than you realised!

As long ago as 1807 a well-known French psychiatrist, Phillipe Pinel, said, 'The primary seat of insanity generally is the region of the stomach and intestines.' What a clever man! But despite many physicians over the centuries being aware of the gut–brain connection, scientific research in this area is still in its infancy.

If you have mental health problems that you intuitively feel are caused by your body chemistry going wrong and not by stress, grief or trauma, this section of the book is for you. I appreciate that this information may sound radical if you have never considered that your gut could affect your emotions – but it most certainly can.

Mental health issues or brain symptoms?

For the purposes of this book, I have mostly referred to depression, anxiety, panic disorder, phobias and so on, as 'mental health issues'. However, I'm not entirely comfortable with the term 'mental health', especially if the source of all your bother stems from a physical cause. If mental health issues arise from a physical cause due to an imbalance in body chemistry, they should surely be referred to as 'brain symptoms' and not 'mental health issues'.

Let me give you an example of why I feel so strongly about this. Let's say someone has an undiagnosed gluten sensitivity. Gluten intolerance can cause depression and anxiety (Busby et al 2018) and so the patient would be labelled as a person with mental health problems. But why? Surely the correct label is 'brain symptoms' because they result from an allergic response. And, once gluten is removed from the diet, the mental health symptoms will probably disappear, proving it's not a mental health problem at all.

A few years ago, I read a wonderful book called *The Missing Diagnosis* (1985) by C Orian Truss. He started his career as a cardiologist but later specialised in helping people with mental health problems that were not being helped by the standard medical approach. His patients had been labelled as neurotic by the medical profession but Truss believed that the cause of many mental illnesses was *Candida albicans*. This is a yeast that overgrows in the digestive tract of some people with gut dysbiosis. Truss demonstrated that *Candida* overgrowth triggers a storm of reactions that affect many organs, including the brain. When Truss helped his patients correct their gut dysbiosis and *Candida* overgrowth, their mental health symptoms vanished, leading him to believe his patients did not have any mental health problems and were, in fact, suffering from brain symptoms because of that *Candida* overgrowth. Truss specialised in *Candida* as a cause of brain symptoms, but I believe there are plenty more biological causes that need exploring.

I may be labouring the point, but it feels important to me to distinguish between mental health issues that have a physical cause and those that are an emotional response to trauma, stress and grief. What I had seen in myself and in my clients convinced me that Truss was right and that some mental illnesses have been wrongly labelled. So, from then on, when consulting my clients I have always referred to their mental health symptoms as brain symptoms.

I feel it's important to know the cause of your mental health problems. For the sake of your identity and peace of mind, it's important to understand that the origin of your brain symptoms could be physical. The other reason is so that you can get the right treatment. The correct diagnosis of any illness is essential to recovery. Without it you are just stabbing in the dark.

'Mental health problems' implies you should be laid on a psychiatrist's couch. But if your symptoms have a physical cause, you could talk about your emotions until the cows come home and still not feel any better!

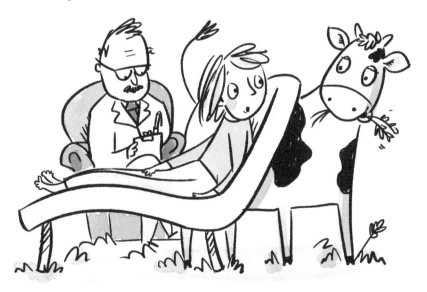

What if it's physical, not psychological?

What if you're biochemically different to people who don't suffer with their mental health? What if you could have tests to discover exactly what your biochemical differences are and then take nutritional supplements to correct your differences? Well, you can! Because I've done it, and so have my clients and lots of other people (Walsh et al 2004).

We've been led to believe that mental illness is directly related to the mind, but I don't believe this is always the case. There are lots of ways in which physical disturbances can cause mental health issues. Let me give you a few examples:

» B12 deficiency can cause depression and apathy (Sahu et al 2022)
» vitamin D deficiency can cause depression (Akpinar & Karadag 2022)
» B3 deficiency has been linked to schizophrenia (Periyasamy et al 2019)
» copper overload can cause depression and anxiety
» food intolerances have been linked to psychosis (Rippere 1984).

If you presented these symptoms to your doctor, there's a chance they would prescribe pharmaceuticals or refer you for counselling, neither of which would help you if the cause of your mental health issues is a vitamin deficiency or a food intolerance.

I think modern psychiatry is missing a trick! In my experience, GPs and psychiatrists rarely run tests to check for basic biochemical imbalances in patients with mental health problems before prescribing antidepressants or anti-anxiety medication. In how many other areas of medicine do doctors prescribe drugs without first running tests? It makes more sense to me to first discover what exactly is causing a client's brain symptoms.

It's a tragedy when mental health symptoms are misdiagnosed as psychiatric when the cause is biological. It leads to the patient feeling neurotic and utterly despairing of ever feeling well again.

The tricky thing is that psychological stress leads to an almost identical clinical picture as mental health issues caused by physical disturbances. So, how do you or your doctor know if the cause of your mental health problems is reactive (resulting from external circumstances) or endogenous (having an internal cause or origin)?

The answer in my practice is to start with my three-point plan and monitor my client's physical and mental health. We soon begin to see what's working and what the impact of good nutrition can be on the mind.

This is usually when I'd recommend a handful of private blood tests to hopefully pinpoint exactly what the problem is. I'll be discussing some of the more common conditions that can cause brain symptoms in a later chapter. All of these can be tested for and treated and none of them can be cured by antidepressants or counselling. I know antidepressants have helped millions of people worldwide, but the majority of my clients haven't felt any better when taking medication and that's why they've come to me – to try a different approach.

SSRI antidepressant medication emerged from the discovery that an imbalance in neurotransmitters is associated with mental illness. For example, low serotonin is associated with depression and elevated noradrenaline can cause anxiety. But unfortunately, there's an important question that modern science has forgotten to ask: why do some people have an imbalance in neurotransmitters? To answer that we need to go right back to basics.

The raw materials that produce and govern neurotransmitters are vitamins, minerals and amino acids. For example, the production of serotonin requires tryptophan and B6. The production of gamma-aminobutyric acid (GABA) needs zinc and B6, and the production of dopamine needs folate and iron (Tardy et al 2020). It surely can't be a coincidence that three common deficiencies that are flagged up in my clients' blood tests are iron, zinc and B6. If at all possible, surely it makes more sense to correct the imbalance at source with nutrients that are natural to the body, rather than introducing pharmaceutical drugs that are foreign to the body and come with a long list of possible side effects?

We must also consider why some people seem predisposed to an imbalance in neurotransmitters. I think the answer lies in epigenetics. A person's environment, such as their diet, stress levels and exposure to chemicals such as pesticides, can all affect the expression of their genes (Weinhold 2006). This explains why one identical twin can manifest a disease while the other twin is healthy. It depends on their lifestyle. Your genes load the gun but it's your lifestyle choices that pull the trigger.

Many mental health conditions run in families (NIH 2013). This can make people feel as if they are doomed to inherit the same problems, but I don't think this is the case. You may have a genetic predisposition but it's possible to correct your body chemistry. This is the case in my family. After I was diagnosed with copper overload and pyrrole disorder, I advised my mum to get tested because she's also prone to panic attacks. And sure enough, she had copper overload and pyrrole disorder. We'll never know for sure, but I'd be willing to bet that we inherited this from my granny, who also suffered. So, although I inherited this condition, it's by no means set in stone. Now that blood tests have diagnosed exactly what's gone wrong with my body chemistry, I've been able to correct it with nutrients.

As we go through the book, I'll be discussing various conditions and deficiencies that I've come across in my practice that I believe have contributed to my clients' brain symptoms, and explaining how I've treated them with my three-point plan.

The three-point plan and mental health

Over the years, many of my clients (mostly women) have suffered from a combination of gut dysbiosis, anxiety and depression. As they follow my three-point plan, both their digestive symptoms and their mental health symptoms improve, implying to me that the two are connected. I think one of the reasons my clients' gut and brain symptoms improve at a similar rate is due to absorption. Nature provided us with our own vitamin-making machine, our gut microbiome. But when dysbiosis occurs, it hinders the gut's vitamin-making and absorption abilities, leading to deficiencies. But, as digestive function improves, my clients are once again able to absorb the vitamins and minerals from their food and the deficiencies are corrected.

Modern medicine has divided illness into different systems: the nervous system, endocrine system, digestive system, etc – and doctors specialise in each of these different areas. However, this method overlooks the fact that all the organs and systems work together and are interdependent. Take psychiatry, for example. This is a classic example of a stand-alone area of medicine. Modern psychiatry doesn't consider the connection between the brain and other systems of the body, although there have been many scientific studies linking psychiatric disorders to a physical cause. Fortunately, some doctors and researchers have dedicated their careers to researching the link between nutrition and mental health. Abram Hoffer, Carl Pfeiffer and William Walsh are pioneers in this area and I recommend looking up their books.

I will be recommending lots of books, but if you were to buy only one, make it *Nutrient Power* by William J Walsh (2012). In his 30-plus years of research, he has collected hundreds of thousands of blood samples of mentally ill patients. It was here that I first read about copper overload, which led me to test my own levels and was the final piece of the jigsaw in my healing journey. I have since recommended this test to some of my clients who, like me, have seen great results by lowering their copper levels, simply by taking a few vitamin supplements.

Most of my clients see an improvement when they follow my three-point plan. That's because eating clean, taking supportive supplements and having a less stressful lifestyle corrects nutritional deficiencies, reduces toxic load, rebalances the gut microbiome and reduces inflammation – all of which benefit mental health.

I realise that nutrition may sound like a novel approach, but biological treatment for mental health issues is becoming more common. Biological psychiatrists are still in the minority, but fortunately it's now recognised that there are many physical causes of mental health problems.

Psychobiotics

The gut–brain connection is a relatively new area of research. In recent years, laboratories have been set up worldwide that are researching the link between gut health and psychological and neurological conditions. Studies are linking the bacteria in our gut microbiome to a wide range of conditions, including anxiety, depression, autism, Parkinson's, Alzheimer's and schizophrenia. Regular patterns are emerging from this research. For example, one trial showed that patients with schizophrenia all had the same strain of 'bad' bacteria in their faeces (Xiang et al 2022). So, scientists testing a variety of faeces knew who had schizophrenia and who didn't just from the presence of this one bacterium. These findings are exciting because if we can pinpoint exactly which bacteria relate to which mental health issue, it might one day be possible to make a range of probiotic-type supplements that all target different mental health issues.

Researchers have coined the term 'psychobiotics' to describe the treatment they're researching in this field. Psychobiotics are drugs containing live bacteria, such as probiotics, which interact with gut bacteria and the gut–brain axis and produce health benefits in patients suffering from psychiatric illness. In trials, symptoms of depression and anxiety are being alleviated, suggesting that the effects of psychobiotics are comparable to the effects of antidepressant medication (Sarkar et al 2016).

Psychobiotics are still a long way off being marketed as pharmaceutical drugs, but don't despair – you can improve your own gut microbiome. You can correct gut dysbiosis and make your tummy a happy, healthy place. Following my three-point plan should redress the balance of bacteria in your gut. You'll know if you're on the right track because your symptoms should start improving within a few weeks.

Interesting titbit

A pivotal study found that mice with gut dysbiosis had an exaggerated reaction to stress. Their abnormal stress response was reversible through psychobiotics, which recolonised their gut microbiome (Studo et al 2004).

Brain structure

Did you know that emotional trauma can cause structural changes to the brain? Perhaps you have seen the infamous picture of the two toddlers' brain scans (Perry 2002)? One toddler had been abused and neglected and the other toddler had been nurtured in a loving environment. The toddler who suffered abuse had a significantly smaller brain than the loved one. It stands to reason that a smaller than average brain must produce brain symptoms. After all, an enlarged heart or an underdeveloped liver would probably produce some kind of symptoms. Similar structural changes have been seen in the brain scans of Romanian orphans who suffered neglect as infants (Chugani et al 2001). More subtle structural brain changes have also been observed in people who have suffered emotional trauma. These changes have been observed in the amygdala, hippocampus and prefrontal cortex areas of the brain (Bremner 2006).

Adverse childhood experiences are commonly linked to mental illness later in life. However, this label of mental illness doesn't sit comfortably with me. I think it implies that these people can't get over their past trauma, or that they're depressed about what happened to them. It suggests that their feelings are within their control, which could make the sufferer feel neurotic and extremely frustrated with themselves when, in fact, they have suffered a type of structural brain damage that is being misdiagnosed as an emotional problem.

The ramifications of this are beyond the scope of this book, but I strongly believe that these people should *not* be labelled as mentally ill. They are suffering from brain symptoms. This is why I would love to see a brand-new approach to the treatment of mental health because it seems unlikely that talking therapy and antidepressants alone could cure these people when their brain has suffered structural changes as a result of emotional trauma (see studies cited in Walsh 2012).

> **Interesting titbit**
> Another structural change to the brain has been spotted by Professor Michael Crawford, co-author (with David E Marsh) of *The Shrinking Brain* (2023). He says the size of the human brain has shrunk by 20 per cent. Yikes! IQ scores are also falling and mental illness is rising. We're actually regressing as a species!

Brain symptoms and you

Next, let's explore how likely is it that your brain symptoms have a physical cause. Read through the following questions and see how many of them apply to you.

» Have you used birth control pills or HRT?
» Have you had multiple pregnancies?
» Do you have digestive disturbances?
» Are you prone to allergies?
» Do you have food sensitivities?
» Do you have low alcohol tolerance?
» Have you had multiple courses of antibiotics?
» Are you prone to frequent colds and infections?
» Have you taken immunosuppressant drugs?
» Have you had a poor diet?
» Do you experience regular fatigue?
» Have you had times of chronic stress?
» Have you experienced physical or emotional trauma or abuse?
» Does mental illness run in your family?
» Do you find that antidepressants and tranquillisers don't help you?
» Did you have health issues in your early years?

If you answered yes to five or more of these questions, I would say there's a possibility your brain symptoms could be attributed to a physical cause.

Anxiety and gut dysbiosis

It's completely normal to feel slight anxiety regarding unpleasant digestive symptoms. A common anxiety is being away from home and needing to quickly find a toilet. That's enough to send anyone into a panic! But the anxiety I'd like to discuss is much more than rational feelings of concern. It's a feeling of high anxiety that expresses itself physically, with symptoms such as an elevated heart rate, sweating, disorientation, hyperventilating or even a full-blown panic attack. Of course, these intense feelings of anxiety will only apply to a small percentage of people reading this book, but I've seen it in too many of my clients, not to mention the apparent link between digestive troubles and high anxiety. Clients often describe it as feeling the physical symptoms of anxiety but not actually feeling worried about anything in particular – as if the trigger is physical, not mental. Clients have told me they were sweating and trembling but weren't sure why. There's a definite link between gut problems and anxiety, and I believe one can trigger the other.

It's easy to understand that a panic attack could trigger symptoms such as diarrhoea, and I'm sure most people can relate to this feeling. After all, almost all of us have experienced diarrhoea when feeling nervous about something. But what's more unusual is to be sitting at home feeling perfectly relaxed when, out of the blue, unpleasant feelings of intense anxiety start washing over you.

Some of my clients have managed to identify a food type that triggers their anxious feelings. Keeping up to date with your food journal can help you with this. Sugar was the most common food my clients identified as their anxiety/panic trigger. This is probably because sugary foods cause blood sugar levels to rise within minutes of eating. Alcohol is another common cause. Another trigger can be foods you are allergic or intolerant to. This can cause a rapid heartbeat, which may trigger anxious feelings. But for many people, the cause of their anxious feelings was much less obvious than a link to any particular food and therefore baffling and hard to control.

Anxiety can make you feel as though you're going crazy as if at any moment something in your brain could 'snap' and you'll be carted away in a straitjacket! This isn't going to happen. Anxiety isn't your brain malfunctioning. It's a very real biochemical process and not necessarily related to emotional stress or to your personality. It may lead to panic attacks, and panic attacks may lead to agoraphobia, so it's important for you to regain control of your health as soon as you can. The word agoraphobia is based on ancient Greek and it translates as 'fear of the public marketplace'. It's important not to give in to fears of leaving the house because your world can close in on you very quickly. You can lose your confidence in a very short space of time.

This is where brain symptoms that have a physical cause and brain symptoms that have an emotional cause can overlap. Although the anxious feelings may have started out with a physical cause, the fear of the fear compounds and perpetuates the problem. Then it can be tricky to work out the root cause of your anxiety. For this reason, I think it's important to run a few tests to help you understand what initially triggered your anxious feelings, so that you know how to tackle them.

I promise that it's possible to reverse or reduce your anxiety disorder and feel well again. I've seen lots of my clients make life-changing progress. A combination of treating the physical cause through diet and supplements and then dealing with the fear of the fear through counselling can work well.

The stigma of mental illness

In order to destigmatise human emotional health, I think it might be helpful to stop using the term 'mental illness' altogether. Whether the cause of brain symptoms is biological or whether it's emotional, it's all *completely normal*! I would even argue that in some cases it's *completely healthy*. I always remember one of my clients telling me she felt 'doolally' when a health professional diagnosed her with a mental health disorder. This lovely woman had experienced years of abuse from her ex-husband and the prolonged stress had led to her experiencing irritable bowel syndrome, which then led to her being deficient in several vitamins and minerals. On top of all this she was experiencing compulsive behaviours that were interfering with her everyday life. In my opinion, this woman was experiencing normal trauma responses and coping mechanisms. I think it would have been comforting for her to be able to discuss her physical symptoms and brain symptoms with health professionals without them labelling her as mentally ill.

You'll be pleased to know that she made a wonderful recovery. As part of my three-point plan, we healed her digestion, redressed her vitamin deficiencies and incorporated some daily stress-relieving techniques. She found that feeling physically stronger and emotionally calmer helped her to feel less controlled by her compulsive behaviours and she followed her lifelong ambition of becoming a midwife and enrolled at university.

Unfortunately, there's still some stigma surrounding mental illness because some short-sighted people assume mental health issues are a sign of weakness. But everyone I've met with brain symptoms are all extremely strong, resilient and compassionate people.

I understand how embarrassing brain symptoms can feel because I've experienced the humiliating feelings myself. However, it shouldn't feel embarrassing. After all, you wouldn't feel embarrassed about having a dicky heart or a broken leg! Thankfully, this is becoming less and less frequent as more people are speaking openly about their mental health problems. The young royals – William, Catherine, Harry and Meghan – have done sterling work to raise awareness of mental health, as have the singers Lewis Capaldi and George Ezra. The more people who speak openly about their struggle, the more accepting everyone will become.

There have been so many times in the past when I've had a panic attack while out with friends or family and it made me feel so silly. After all, not many people understand the sheer terror of a panic attack. Consequently, to an outsider, it might have seemed as though I was being a drama queen or an attention seeker! Thankfully, I have a very supportive network of people around me who have always done their best to be compassionate and understanding.

I hope you're surrounded by friends, family and professionals who do their best to understand and support you. Keep reminding yourself that your feelings aren't imaginary; they're very real, and for many people, they have a physical cause. It's my sincere wish for you that, as you heal your gut, boost your vitamin and mineral status and bring your body chemistry back into balance, your mental health issues subside.

A true story

A friend of mine used to be a nurse at a psychiatric health hospital in York. One night she was at work and had a bad cold. The pressure in her sinuses became so bad it caused her eardrum to burst, and so her colleagues rang 111. The operator immediately made her an appointment at A&E. She was seen by a male doctor whose manner was extremely rude and offhand. He asked her some odd questions, such as, 'Have you been shoving things down your ears?' When she said no, she had not, he asked her if she imagined the pain in her ears. By this time, my friend was starting to lose her patience and exclaimed, 'Why on earth would I make it up?' The doctor replied, 'Well, it says in these notes that you've come from the mental hospital.' When my friend explained she was a nurse there, the doctor's manner changed; he became professional and polite and treated her with care. However, this experience broke my friend's heart because she couldn't bear to think of her lovely patients being treated with a lack of respect just because they had mental health problems.

Mental health problems can affect anyone. That doctor would do well to remember 'There but for the grace of God go I' and in future show some compassion. Thankfully this kind of small-minded discrimination is seen less and less nowadays. His rudeness seems even more ignorant if we consider the biological process behind mental illness. This doctor had devoted his professional life to correcting biochemical issues, from thyroid problems to heart issues, but where mental health issues were concerned, he mistakenly believed that it was imaginary or a weakness of mind and was oblivious to the fact that the body was malfunctioning, just the same as with any other illness.

I have a story of my own involving a narrow-minded counsellor. In the years prior to my diagnosis of pyrrole disorder and copper overload, I tried every possible form of therapy to help me combat my panic attacks. CBT, psychotherapy, hypnosis... you name it, I've tried it! I've tried every coping technique in the book. I've psycho-analysed myself to within an inch of my life, and the conclusion myself and other professionals came to is that my problem with panic attacks isn't 'in my head' and I don't have any 'issues'. I'm a pretty chilled-out person, and yet the panic attacks persisted. This is what led to my interest in there being a physical cause of many mental health issues.

Bearing all this in mind, many years ago, my then boyfriend and I went to couples counselling. My ex is a nice guy and openly admitted he had some issues he wanted to overcome. But once the counsellor discovered I'd been having occasional panic attacks her entire focus became fixated on me. She was convinced that I was the reason my ex struggled with commitment. He explained that he'd been like this with every woman he'd ever dated, and I explained that I'd tried every therapy going. Still, the counsellor's final diagnosis was basically that I couldn't expect a man to commit to me until I got over my panic attacks. Ouch!

I'm fortunate to have great parents who love me unconditionally, so I've always felt secure and confident in my own skin. And thank goodness for that because the counsellor was suggesting that I would be unlovable until I got a grip of my panic attacks! But, at this stage, no one had ever told me there could be a biological cause; I hadn't worked it out for myself, and I hadn't yet been diagnosed with pyrrole disorder and copper overload. So it left me feeling despairing and frustrated with myself.

My clients with brain symptoms often tell me how angry and frustrated they get with themselves, and it breaks my heart. We've been led to believe mental illness is all in the mind and therefore we should be able to find the mental strength to will ourselves better. But that's not how it works. If you've ever felt cross and frustrated that you couldn't control your brain symptoms, then please stop it right now! Would you get frustrated with yourself if you had cancer and berate yourself for not having the mental strength to make yourself well? Of course you wouldn't. At least, I hope you wouldn't. So please, please don't beat yourself up if you're suffering from brain symptoms.

Interesting titbit
A large-scale study conducted in 2023 (Queensland Brain Institute) reported that one in every two people will struggle with their mental health at some point in their life. You're not on your own.

I'm aware that there are many excellent counsellors, psycho-therapists and psychiatrists, but most of my clients end up coming to me because they haven't been helped by a traditional approach and so, over the years, I've heard a lot of negative stories. I wish I had time to tell you them all because some are almost comical.

I have another disappointing story of my own. Many years ago during a period of debilitating anxiety I was referred to a psychiatric unit for a consultation about what treatments might help me. The doctor there told me the only treatment available at that time was group therapy. This increased my anxiety because I'd never had therapy in a group setting before and so I asked a few questions about how it worked. The doctor said he would go and ask the woman who ran the group therapy sessions to come and answer my questions and hopefully allay my anxieties. But the lady who ran the group took one look at me and vanished! Looking sheepish, the doctor explained that she had recognised me from salsa class and felt it would be unethical to speak to me. I asked how I could go to her talking therapy sessions if she refused to speak to me.

But the doctor just shrugged and no alternative treatment was offered to me. Needless to say, I didn't feel able to attend her group, which left me without help at a time when I really needed it.

This true story highlights the way in which mental illness and physical illness are often treated completely differently. Can you imagine going to A&E with chest pains or a broken leg and the only health professional who could help refuses to speak to you because they recognise you from a public setting? They would probably be struck off! And yet it was considered acceptable to turn me away without treatment during a mental health crisis. Both mental illness and physical illness can be signs that body chemistry isn't working correctly, and I believe both deserve the same care and attention. And yet many people experiencing brain symptoms are left without access to mental health services for one reason or another.

Dear reader, if you have experienced brain symptoms and have ever felt the desire to use your experience to help others, then I urge you to acquire the necessary qualifications. I think that therapists with personal experience of mental health struggles will have a lot to offer their clients. With mental health diagnoses on the rise, your unique skills and first-hand experience are desperately needed.

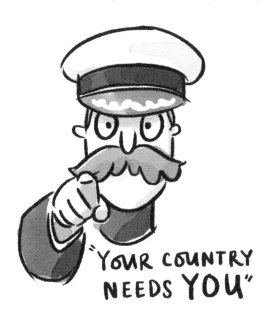

Case study

A nutritionist colleague of mine had a client with depression who had recently moved to a beautiful house surrounded by fields. Within a few months of moving, she changed from being a happy woman with a cheerful disposition to an extremely depressed and tearful one. Her doctor prescribed antidepressants and offered to refer her for counselling, but she intuitively felt that there was nothing wrong with her emotionally, so she began searching for an alternative cure. It was a long and arduous detective journey. The first clue came when her husband inherited a holiday home in France and they spent long periods there. Her depression would always start to lift and then usually return when they went home to the UK. She became convinced she was allergic to something in her house. The second clue came when she realised she felt better during the winter months when the fields around her house were fallow. She finally pieced the puzzle together and realised she was allergic to the pesticides sprayed on the crops. They eventually moved house and her depression permanently lifted.

This is a fascinating case study. How many of us would have had her self-belief that there was nothing wrong emotionally? And her strength of character to continue searching for an environmental or physical cause? I think this was a case of cerebral allergy but unfortunately there isn't a test available that could prove 100 per cent that her self-diagnosis was accurate.

Drug therapy is the modern way of dealing with illness but it doesn't appear to be working because mental and physical diseases are ever increasing. Antidepressants and anti-anxiety medications are useful as a short-term option during periods of extreme stress and depression, but they don't usually solve the underlying problem, so other corrective treatment such as dietary changes and vitamin supplements are a great accompaniment to pharmaceuticals.

There are many physical causes of mental health issues that may not be picked up by your GP, but you will already have an inkling of whether your mental health issues originate from a physical or emotional cause. I always ask my clients why they think they are ill and advise them to trust their gut feeling. More often than not they are right.

Summing up brain health

I hope you aren't feeling too overwhelmed at the end of this chapter. I realise I've thrown a lot of information at you. My aim was to empower you, not overwhelm you. Start by following my three-point plan and see if you feel any reduction in your brain symptoms. If you do, you know you're on the right track. Consult a nutritionist or doctor who can offer you further guidance and refer you for the blood tests I'll be recommending.

I'm not suggesting that digestive troubles and vitamin deficiencies are at the root of every emotional and physical ailment out there, but it's worth being aware of the risk factors and applying the necessary cautions, such as implementing the three-point plan. You have nothing to lose!

I realise that the link between gut health and mental health doesn't have a great deal of scientific evidence to back it up yet. But just because something hasn't been scientifically validated doesn't mean it has been disproven. The one thing we know for sure about scientific evidence is that it's continually evolving, and something that was once scientifically proven is often disproven at a later stage as knowledge and technology advance. So, for this reason, I always listen to anecdotal evidence. Perhaps a more dignified term that means the same thing is 'empirical evidence', which is defined as anything provable or verifiable by experience. There are many real-life stories which show that people have improved their digestive health and nutritional status and consequently their mental health has improved. We're fortunate to have forums for just about every ailment under the sun, so do your research.

If the day comes when Western medicine and other forms of therapy such as nutritional therapy can work together in harmony and with respect, that's the day we'll see true healing take place. One last thing I'd like to say at the close of this chapter is that I understand how truly awful it is to suffer from brain symptoms and to feel out of control of your body and emotions. So, I sincerely hope that you will benefit from a diet and supplement programme, just like I have, along with countless others. Know that you're not alone. There are thousands of people fighting their own personal battles and having to make changes and sacrifices for the sake of their health. You can be free. Don't give up hope.

Chapter 4

Conditions that may be causing your brain symptoms

In this chapter, we're searching for a biological cause of your brain symptoms. These conditions often go hand in hand with gut dysbiosis because it can cause malabsorption, which then causes vitamin and mineral deficiencies. Deficiencies affect the biochemical processes within the body and brain. This is why I believe that your focus must always be on gut health as a cause or contributor to your brain symptoms.

All of the conditions discussed in this chapter can cause brain symptoms. Unfortunately, they are often overlooked or misdiagnosed. All of the following conditions can be diagnosed with the appropriate tests, but be aware you would probably have to pay to have these tests done privately. Each of the conditions can be corrected by a clean diet, lifestyle changes and the correct nutritional supplements. Unfortunately, doctors rarely prescribe vitamin and mineral supplements because a pharmaceutical approach is favoured. But there are private GPs out there who can support you.

These are doctors who have continued training at their own expense after graduating from medical school. The doctor I consulted for my diagnosis of pyrrole disorder and copper overload was wonderful. She had travelled to the US to study at the Walsh Institute. William J Walsh is a doctor, scientist and author of more than 200 scientific articles. He has devoted his career to helping people with mental illness, and amassed thousands of patient blood samples from which he has identified certain biochemical differences in people experiencing brain symptoms. He has developed natural treatments that have helped his patients to recover their health. It was his book *Nutrient Power* that led to my personal diagnosis. This approach to treating disease is called orthomolecular medicine.

Orthomolecular medicine

The term orthomolecular medicine was coined by Linus Pauling (biochemist, author and Nobel prize winner). It describes the treatment of disease using nutrients. An orthomolecular approach to health treats the cause of disease by looking at the optimal concentrations of vitamins and minerals needed for full health. Vitamins and minerals are the raw materials our body needs to function; they are essential for good health and even a mild deficiency will lead to the body malfunctioning. For example, vitamin B3 plays an important role in more than 500 reactions in the body! Five hundred! So you can see why a deficiency in B3 would cause some unpleasant symptoms.

An orthomolecular approach identifies the vitamin and mineral deficiencies that are causing your ill health through testing of blood and urine and then uses nutrient therapy to normalise vitamin and mineral levels. Let me give you a few examples of health conditions linked to deficiencies. A deficiency in calcium has been linked to osteoporosis. A deficiency in B12 can cause DNA damage and has also been linked to anxiety and depression. A deficiency in vitamin A has been linked to lung cancer. A B6 deficiency is linked to pancreatic cancer. Vitamin D deficiency is linked to colorectal cancer, breast cancer tumours and depression. A deficiency in iodine has been linked to breast cancer. A deficiency in B3 has been linked to schizophrenia. I could go on, but I'm sure you get the picture of how important your vitamin and mineral status is. But how many of us regularly check our vitamin status? And how many GPs investigate vitamin and mineral deficiencies as the cause of mental and physical illness? No one ever got cancer because of a deficiency in chemotherapy, but many people have developed it due to vitamin and mineral deficiencies. (See Venturelli et al 2021, Rappaport 2017, Sangle et al 2020 and Cao et al 2018 for research studies on some of these links.)

It's widely known and accepted that a deficiency in folate can cause birth defects in children and nowadays pregnant women take folic acid as a matter of course. But the doctor who discovered this connection was ridiculed for being too simplistic and it was many years before his discovery was accepted as fact. Unfortunately, Western medicine still scoffs at the importance of orthomolecular medicine and a pharmaceutical approach to disease is nearly always favoured over a nutritional approach. I think the only way we can change this paradigm is for everyone to start taking responsibility for their own health.

Adapt your diet and lifestyle and search for the root cause of your ailments. If this approach doesn't work for you, then accept pharmaceutical drugs, but not before. No amount of medication can save you from a bad diet, so it's important to take accountability for the lifestyle you're choosing.

It's becoming more accepted that nutrition is a crucial factor in cardiology, endocrinology and gastroenterology and I think there's compelling evidence that nutrition also plays an important role in mental health and, as such, deserves further research (Sarris et al 2015).

As you read about the following conditions, you'll notice that many of them influence neurotransmitters. These are chemical messengers that help control heart rate, blood pressure, emotions, stress response, hormone regulation and digestion. Examples of neurotransmitters include glutamate, GABA, serotonin, dopamine, histamine, epinephrine (aka adrenalin) and norepinephrine. I think we need to take a broader look at the various neurotransmitters because it's possible to manipulate them naturally without the use of selective serotonin reuptake inhibitors (SSRIs).

Take your time reading this next section and see if you can relate to any of the symptoms I mention. They could give you a clue as to which, if any, of the conditions you're suffering from. If any resonate with you, your next step could be to organise the appropriate tests to get a definite diagnosis. Some of my clients have had more than one condition. This is quite common. So, bear it in mind as you read on.

Vitamin and mineral deficiencies

I think that testing for vitamin and mineral deficiencies should be the first port of call for *any* illness – but especially mental illness. I recommend always looking for the cause of your ailment rather than treating the symptoms. Vitamins and minerals are responsible for hundreds of important bodily functions and so deficiencies interrupt the workings of the body.

Ideally, we would all be testing our full range of vitamins and minerals every couple of years but unfortunately this would prove very expensive. And so, below, I have briefly listed the deficiencies I've most regularly seen in my clients. I haven't gone into great detail here because I discuss vitamins in more detail later in the book. But I wanted to make the point here that I believe vitamin and mineral deficiencies are one of the main contributors to misdiagnosis of mental illness.

Here are the vitamins and minerals I most commonly test for, but there are many more. If you consult a nutritional therapist, they will go through an in-depth questionnaire that will indicate which vitamins and minerals you're deficient in, and this may give you some guidance regarding which blood tests to choose.

B6 deficiency

B6 is required for more than 100 chemical processes in the body, and it plays an important role in brain function. It's essential in the synthesis of the neurotransmitters serotonin, dopamine and GABA.

Signs of deficiency include: irritability, depression, psychosis, pyrrole disorder, OCD, insomnia, muscle weakness, sore tongue, cracks in the corner of the mouth, fatigue and skin rashes (McCulloch 2023).

Vitamin D deficiency

Vitamin D is sometimes called the sunshine vitamin because the body makes it when we're exposed to sunlight. You can also find it in oily fish, red meat and egg yolks. It's one of the most common nutritional deficiencies in the UK (due to our low levels of exposure to bright sunlight), which is probably why it's one of the few vitamins tested for and prescribed by GPs. Vitamin D deficiency is associated with depression, ADHD, poor immune function, fatigue, poor sleep, back pain, hair loss and schizophrenia, plus alterations in GABA and dopamine (Cui et al 2021).

Zinc deficiency

Zinc is an essential mineral found in many foods. Zinc deficiency is common in people with mental health problems. This could be because many people with mental health conditions have high oxidative stress (see below), which depletes zinc. Zinc is needed to maintain the blood–brain barrier, which stops harmful chemicals from entering the brain. Signs and symptoms of zinc deficiency include poor immunity, hormone imbalance, anxiety, depression, loss of smell and taste, poor wound healing, skin rashes, low libido, lethargy, irritability, aggression, copper overload and low GABA (Watson 2019).

Magnesium deficiency

Magnesium plays an essential role in more than 300 functions in the body. Magnesium deficiency has been linked to reduced serotonin and GABA. Signs and symptoms of magnesium deficiency include apathy, stress, depression, fatigue, sleep issues and aches and pains. My clients regularly present with all these symptoms. The good news is that taking a magnesium supplement can reduce these unpleasant symptoms within a few weeks (Arnarson 2023).

Folate – friend or foe?

Both folate deficiency and folate overload are related to brain symptoms. For this reason, it's a supplement I wouldn't recommend unless my client had a blood test to check their folate levels. Folate supplements can worsen brain symptoms in people who under-methylate (see the section on methylation below), and so these people must avoid folate supplements and any other supplements containing folate (Walsh 2012).

I recently spoke to a nutritionist colleague who had a bad experience when she took a folic acid supplement, plus a multivitamin containing folic acid. This was many years ago, before she qualified as a nutritionist, and so she didn't understand the implications. She had been suffering with depression at that time and the folic acid had made her feel so terrible she couldn't get out of bed. Fortunately, she's now fully recovered. Her experience has made me doubly cautious. I recommend that you treat folic acid with caution until you've been tested.

When grains became mass produced, all the goodness was lost during the refining process and so folic acid was added. But if you're prone to undermethylation, this could exacerbate your mental health symptoms. Mental illness increased with the onset of 'fortifying' foods – in particular the fortifying of wheat in the 1940s (National Library of Medicine 2003; Dohan 1966). This could be a coincidence but it's worth considering.

However, in some people a folate deficiency has been linked to depression, and taking a folate supplement has made them feel better (Godfrey et al 1990). In my experience, many more people benefit from folate than the small number who react badly to it.

Elevated copper levels

Copper is a mineral found throughout the body and has many important functions. But some people (more often women) have a genetic inability to regulate their copper levels, and this results in them having more than they need. This usually has a negative impact on mental health because copper overload negatively affects neurotransmitter function. It can lower dopamine levels and increase norepinephrine in the brain. Elevated norepinephrine is linked to schizophrenia, depression, panic disorder, severe anxiety and ADHD. Correcting copper overload with the correct nutrients will bring down norepinephrine levels (Walsh 2012).

Copper overload is usually hereditary, which could explain why mental health problems often run in families. Females with high copper levels tend to feel a worsening of brain symptoms when they take hormones such as the contraceptive pill or hormone replacement therapy (HRT). This is because these medications increase copper levels. In my practice I've found copper overload to be more common than copper deficiency.

Some of the conditions we'll be looking at go hand in hand. This is often because they stem from the same vitamin deficiencies. People with elevated copper tend to have low levels of zinc. Low levels of zinc are associated with pyrrole disorder and also oxidative stress. Many people are diagnosed with all three conditions.

Signs and symptoms

Elevated copper can cause depression (Totten et al 2023), particularly post-partum depression, hormone changes, hyperactivity, learning difficulties, skin sensitivity to tags in clothes or rough fabric, intolerance to oestrogen or birth control pills, onset during puberty/pregnancy/menopause, white spots on fingernails, ringing in the ears, sensitivity to shellfish, high anxiety, PMT, poor immunity, sleep problems, low dopamine activity, elevated norepinephrine and adrenaline, diarrhoea, fatigue, headaches. It also causes a deficiency in glutathione (a powerful antioxidant).

Risk factors

Elevated copper levels are often hereditary. Copper can be found in unfiltered water and in food such as shellfish, organ meats, potatoes and wholegrains. Copper IUDs might also contribute. Zinc deficiency stops excess copper being excreted from the body.

Treatment

Zinc, manganese, glutathione, vitamins B3, B6, C, E. Start on a low dose of zinc and build up gradually to prevent too much copper being excreted at once, which could worsen brain symptoms.

Testing

One of my favourite tests when searching for a biological cause for brain symptoms is a hair mineral analysis, which you can order yourself and do at home. At the time of writing (2024) a test costs around £150. It shows levels of copper and zinc. High levels of copper and low levels of zinc are quite common in my clients with anxiety and depression.

Another great test is a combined one for serum copper, plasma zinc, vitamin D, RBC magnesium and ceruloplasmin. At the time of writing, it costs £125 and I believe it's money well worth spending, but you'd need a doctor's referral. See References and resources and the chapter on testing for more details.

It's helpful to look at the copper/zinc ratio in the body. The UK's recommended reference range for copper is 12–26 µmol/L. However, the doctor I consulted said that, in her experience, lower than 12 is often necessary to relieve brain symptoms. And similarly, the recommended reference range for zinc is 9.6–20.5 µmol/L but 9.6 is too low to see a reduction in symptoms for some people, so I recommend aiming for at least 15 µmol/L.

Case study

Symptoms: Depression, anxiety, weight gain, underactive thyroid.

My client, a 37-year-old female, experienced a decline in health that coincided with the birth of her only child five years previously. She had post-partum depression, which had lessened over time but never completely went away. She had been diagnosed with an underactive thyroid two years previously. She also complained of weight gain and anxiety.

I recommended a hair mineral analysis, which showed slightly raised levels of cadmium. High levels of cadmium have been associated with reduced fertility. My client had been trying for another baby for two years, so there's a possibility the two are related. High levels of cadmium are also associated with smoking. My client had smoked for a few years as a teenager but not since then.

The hair mineral analysis also showed low levels of zinc and high levels of copper. When a woman is pregnant, copper levels in the blood increase and remain elevated for a month or two after giving birth. For some people who have high levels of copper to begin with, the excess copper during pregnancy can cause post-partum depression (Chen et al 2023). This was most likely the cause of my client's post-partum depression.

I think all women should supplement with zinc, B6 and omega 3 while pregnant to avoid copper-related post-partum depression. Food cravings during pregnancy can be a sign of mineral deficiency and an indicator to take a few supportive supplements.

My three-point plan recommendations for my client were...

» **Dietary changes:** Follow the recommendations as laid out in this book, and avoid all stimulants.
» **Lifestyle changes:** I thought some form of exercise would be beneficial, so she started going to local aerobics classes. I also recommended she take time for relaxation, but she struggled to incorporate this recommendation.
» **Supplements:**
  › Zinc helps to support the thyroid, plays an important role in regulation of insulin and lowers copper levels. Zinc is also good for lowering toxic mineral levels, including cadmium. Zinc has helped to reduce brain symptoms in most of my clients.
  › Selenium, as it plays a role in thyroid health, is an antioxidant and supports robust mental health.
  › B6 works with zinc to lower copper levels and also supports robust mental health.

› Omega 3 is an anti-inflammatory and reduces symptoms of depression (Grosso 2014).
› Vitamin C, which rebalances the gut microbiome, reduces oxidative stress and carries toxic minerals out of the body.
› 5-HTP helps to reduce depression.

» **Follow-up:** My client was feeling much better overall. Her mood had lightened, she had more energy and had lost a few pounds in weight. She also mentioned that she'd had a strong body odour for the past few years but that had lessened since she'd been following the three-point plan. This could be due to the detoxification effects of the plan.

We stayed in contact for a year and during that time her symptoms continued to improve. She stuck with the three-point plan, including the supplements, for more than six months. She then transitioned to a lower maintenance programme of supplements and reintroduced a few grains back into her diet. She continued to feel well and pretty much symptom free. I recommended doing another hair mineral analysis, but I think that because she was feeling so much better she couldn't justify the expense.

Pyrrole disorder

Pyrrole disorder is one of the conditions I was diagnosed with later in life, after years of struggling with panic disorder. Abram Hoffer defined the condition in 1958 when he noticed elevated levels of kryptopyrroles in the urine samples of his schizophrenic patients. Kryptopyrroles bind to B6 and zinc, resulting in these essential nutrients being excreted in urine. So people who have excessive pyrroles end up with deficiencies in B6 and zinc, which can result in a range of psychiatric disorders. This may be because zinc and B6 play an essential role in the production of serotonin, dopamine, melatonin and GABA. Low levels of these neurotransmitters in the brain may lead to depression and anxiety (Walsh 2012).

Signs and symptoms

Anxiety, ADHD, autism, bipolar disorder, panic disorder, addictions, Tourette's, OCD, schizophrenia, IBS, pot belly, morning nausea, motion sickness, gluten sensitivity, crowded upper front teeth, joint pain in knees, strong reactions to medications, white flecks on fingernails, joint aches, fatigue, upper abdominal pain, low iron and/or ferritin levels, cold hands and feet, allergies and intolerances, irregular menstruation, severe PMT, having lookalike female relatives who suffer with similar mental health problems, low serotonin, adrenal exhaustion, feeling dependent on one person for security, stretch marks, sensitivity to bright lights and loud noises, pale skin, bad breath and body odour, eczema, psoriasis, thinning hair, prematurely grey hair, headaches, miscarriage of male babies (Walsh 2012).

Risk factors

Pyrrole disorder may be genetically inherited and can also be caused by physical and emotional stressors such as grief and the overuse of antibiotics. More recent research suggests that kryptopyrroles are produced by the bad bacteria found in gut dysbiosis (Rigoni 2020). So, healing the gut will hopefully correct the root cause of pyrrole disorder.

Treatment with supplements (see also Chapter 9)

» Zinc
» B6 (P5P)
» Manganese: because manganese is depleted when zinc is taken at high levels.
» Quercetin: aids the absorption of zinc.
» B3: aids recovery from pyrrole disorder.
» Vitamin C: supports adrenal glands that have been exhausted by pyrrole disorder.
» Glutathione and selenium: to reduce oxidative stress.

People with pyrrole disorder often feel nauseous in the morning so may have to wait until the afternoon before taking supplements. After three months of taking the above supplements, your anxiety levels should have decreased.

Testing

A simple urine test that can be done at home is available from various labs. See the Resources section. At the time of writing, a urine kryptopyrrole test costs £63. Stop taking all supplements for a week before testing. Copper overload and pyrrole disorder often go hand in hand, so I don't recommend testing one without the other.

Oxidative stress

Perhaps you've heard of free radicals? They're unstable molecules found in your body that damage your cells, causing illness and ageing. Lifestyle factors such as smoking, alcohol, pesticides and a diet high in carbohydrates accelerate the production of free radicals.

Antioxidants are helpful chemicals which lessen or prevent the effects of free radicals. Antioxidants are found in fruits, vegetables, turmeric, green tea, the vitamins C and E, and the minerals selenium and zinc.

When your body doesn't have enough antioxidants to keep things in check it allows free radicals to go rogue! They run wild around your body damaging as many cells as possible! This is called oxidative stress. Oxidative stress has been linked to mental illness, diabetes, heart disease, Parkinson's disease, Alzheimer's and cancer. I'd like to bet that the majority of people eating a Western diet have more free radicals than they have antioxidants!

Oxidative stress goes hand in hand with pyrrole disorder and also with copper overload.

This is because oxidative stress depletes zinc and B6.

Oxidative stress can also cause undermethylation and vice versa. You can probably see why the conditions I mention are all linked and why some people are diagnosed with more than one condition.

The brain is highly susceptible to oxidative stress, so it's not surprising that it's implicated in a range of mental illnesses, including depression, anxiety and schizophrenia (Salim 2014).

Oxidative stress can upset digestion because it destroys digestive enzymes. These enzymes play an essential role in digesting your food, so a lack of them hinders complete breakdown of the food you eat, causing digestive issues (Sherman 2023).

Signs and symptoms
Fatigue, brain fog, anxiety, depression, headache, sensitivity to noise, accelerated ageing, unstable blood sugar levels.

Risk factors
Emotional and physical stress, metabolic dysfunction, inflammation, poor diet, smoking, alcohol, pesticides.

Treatment
Highly coloured vegetables: these are full of antioxidants. A concentrated cherry juice called Active Edge Cherry Active is one of my faves! It's chock full of antioxidants (see Resources). It works well on linseed porridge and pancakes.

Vitamin B6, selenium, vitamin E, zinc, glutathione, vitamin C: these nutrients provide neuroprotection of the brain from oxidative injury (Lee et al 2020).

Tests

» A glutathione test (see Resources).

Case study
A woman in her early twenties consulted me after her GP diagnosed her with irritable bowel syndrome. Her main symptoms were reflux, indigestion and occasional diarrhoea after eating – all classic signs

of gut dysbiosis. The other symptoms she presented with were high anxiety, which she chose not to take medication for; acne, which she had previously taken antibiotics for, and fatigue. She looked extremely pale and had visible stretch marks on her skin, both of which can indicate zinc deficiency. She also had crowded upper front teeth, which can be a sign of pyrrole disorder.

Her main concern was irritable bowel syndrome, so she began by implementing my dietary recommendations and started taking a probiotic and a digestive enzyme. I didn't recommend any lifestyle changes because she was passionate about yoga and felt it helped her anxiety, so she did 20 minutes of yoga on most mornings. She quickly saw improvements in her digestion, and as is often the way, commented that her anxiety levels felt a little better too. I then broached the subject of a biological cause of her anxiety and recommended she test herself for copper overload, pyrrole disorder and oxidative stress. She couldn't justify the expense of all three, so I recommended she tested for copper overload and pyrrole disorder because a diagnosis for those conditions pretty much guarantees high oxidative stress. Sure enough, her test results showed elevated kryptopyrroles and copper.

We then added zinc, P5P, vitamin C, glutathione, manganese and selenium to her supplement regimen. She was compliant with the three-point plan and saw big improvements in all her symptoms. The improvements in her digestion were almost immediate but the brain symptoms took a little longer. After three months she said she felt noticeably less anxious, and after six months she said she was feeling the best she'd felt since she was a child. We pared back her supplement regimen slightly and she continued to follow my dietary recommendations 90 per cent of the time. I advised her to take a low dose of zinc and P5P on and off for life.

Interestingly, her acne also cleared up, which was a bonus. This is probably because clean eating allowed her body to detox. Plus, zinc and probiotics have proved to be effective treatments for acne, and so the combination of all three led to a dramatic improvement in her skin (Yee et al 2020; Kober & Bowe 2015).

Subclinical pellagra

Pellagra is a B3 (niacin) deficiency. Thankfully, people rarely die from it these days, but I believe mild deficiencies are still causing neuroses. Subclinical pellagra is the developmental phase of pellagra. Some orthodox physicians believe that unless full-blown pellagra is present, there is no deficiency, which unfortunately means subclinical pellagra is rarely diagnosed by modern medicine, but I believe it's causing mental and physical problems for thousands of undiagnosed people. It can be triggered by digestive troubles, which is why it can go hand in hand with gut dysbiosis (Hoffer 1970). B3 is part of the process of forming serotonin from tryptophan (an essential amino acid). Therefore a deficiency can directly impact your production of serotonin.

Signs and symptoms

Diarrhoea, constipation, tummy ache, loss of appetite, depression, anxiety, psychosis, schizophrenia, fatigue, dermatitis, dementia, sores on lips or tongue, nausea, skin pigment changes in sunlight, headaches (Redzic et al 2023).

Risk factors

Hereditary, gut dysbiosis, alcoholism.

Treatment

B3 is the standard treatment for subclinical pellagra. The recommended dietary allowance (RDA) is 16.5 mg, but this is the amount needed to prevent deficiency. If you're already deficient you need more.

Testing

A blood test can detect niacin deficiency.

Methylation

Methyl groups are an essential part of our diet. They are found in foods such as green leafy vegetables, eggs, fish and meat. Methylation is involved in pretty much every biochemical reaction in the body. It's involved in detoxification, immunity, energy production, balancing hormones, it turns off bad genes, it assists in glutathione production, and it helps regulate neurotransmitters such as serotonin and dopamine. Methylation status can even affect someone's personality! For example, the undermethylated person tends to be strong willed, a high achiever, a perfectionist, with OCD tendencies and seasonal allergies. And the overmethylated person is often non-competitive, artistic, very sociable, with high anxiety. Both undermethylation and overmethylation can cause brain symptoms. Read on to see if you can identify with the symptoms of either (Walsh 2012).

Undermethylation

Signs and symptoms

Low serotonin levels, elevated histamine, seasonal allergies, digestive problems, insomnia, chronic depression, seasonal affective disorder (SAD), OCD, rumination about past events, suicidal tendencies, elevated body temperature, calm demeanour but with inner tension, prone to infections, addictive personality, competitive, struggle to concentrate, high libido, low pain tolerance, phobias, social isolation, high homocysteine, heavy metal build-up, adverse reaction to folic acid, good response to antihistamines, adverse reaction to benzodiazepines, good response to SSRIs (Walsh 2012; Deville 2022).

Treatment

» S-adenosyl-L-methionine (SAM-e), vitamins C, B6, E. Zinc, magnesium.
» Avoid a high-protein diet.

Because undermethylated people respond badly to folate, I don't recommend any supplements that may contain it, such as multivitamins or B complex, unless my client has had blood tests diagnosing their methylation status. Folate steals methyl from the body's cells and so prescribing folate to a person who is undermethylated may worsen their brain symptoms.

Overmethylation

Signs and symptoms

Low histamine and an absence of seasonal allergies, excessive dopamine, food sensitivities, oestrogen dominance, low zinc levels, high copper levels, anxiety, panic attacks, depression, paranoia, ADHD, rumination, sleep problems, slow metabolism, prone to food and chemical sensitivities, empathic, artistic, dry eyes, obsessions without compulsive actions, sleep disorders, autoimmune issues, dry skin, frustration, overweight, restless legs, self-harm, intolerance to antihistamines, good response to benzodiazepines, adverse reaction to SSRIs (Deville 2022).

Treatment

Overmethylated people need folic acid, niacinamide (a form of vitamin B3), vitamins B12, B6, C, E, zinc and glutathione. Low folate levels go hand in hand with overmethylation. It's important to avoid folate in the form of methyl folate because the overmethylated person doesn't want any more methyls thank you very much!

In fact, I wouldn't recommend long-term use of methyl folate to anyone regardless of methylation status. Folic acid may be synthetic but it's much more stable.

A diet rich in B vitamins is beneficial. This would include leafy greens, liver, beef, oysters, eggs and sunflower seeds.

Risk factors

Because it's so important to treat the root cause rather than just the symptoms, I'm continually asking myself about the cause of my clients' conditions. Methylation is affected by diet, environment and lifestyle but genetics are usually the dominant factor. For this reason, healthy eating and supplementation will probably need to be a long-term way of life to maintain healthy methylation. My three-point plan gets to the root cause because it heals and seals the gut, corrects nutritional deficiencies, lowers stress levels, balances hormones, detoxifies, reduces oxidative stress and boosts mitochondrial function – all of which promote healthy methylation.

Tests

Methylation profile. See Resources.

High homocysteine

High homocysteine levels can be a cause of brain symptoms and occasionally a cause of digestive symptoms. What follows is a rather long-winded explanation of why I champion homocysteine testing, but bear with me. I've gone into detail because I think it's the most important health test available – not just for people with gut and brain symptoms but for everyone, and I want you to understand its significance.

Homocysteine is an amino acid that affects methylation. Usually, it's safely converted into other substances within the body, but when there's a shortage of B vitamins this conversion can't take place, and homocysteine levels build up to dangerous levels. And when I say dangerous, I mean *really* dangerous. Homocysteine is a biomarker for more than 100 diseases (Smith & Refsum 2021)!

I recommend that everyone should check their homocysteine level because it's an important indicator of your overall health and risk of future disease. A high homocysteine level isn't just associated with disease, it actually *causes* heart disease, strokes, cancer, diabetes, autoimmune disorders, Alzheimer's, Parkinson's, brain symptoms and more.

It's also linked to the impaired metabolism of serotonin, dopamine and noradrenaline, which can cause brain symptoms. Another reason high homocysteine is linked to mental health problems could be because it damages brain cells and nerves. For the full story on homocysteine, I highly recommend you read *The H Factor Solution* (2003) by James Braly and Patrick Holford.

Signs and symptoms

Tiredness, irritable bowel syndrome, anxiety, depression, allergies, unstable weight, inflammatory bowel disease, aches and pains, frequent colds, pale skin, migraines, sleep problems, mental clarity and memory deterioration, arthritis, asthma or eczema, stomach ulcers, chronic fatigue syndrome, autoimmune disease, family history of heart disease, strokes, Alzheimer's, cancer and depression, miscarriage (Braly & Holford 2003).

Risk factors

Stress and trauma, gut dysbiosis, poor diet, high coffee intake, smoking, excessive alcohol intake, rarely exercising, genetics, being a vegan or vegetarian.

Treatment

The good news is that high levels of homocysteine are easy to correct. All that's needed is a daily supplement containing B2, B6, folic acid, B12 and zinc. My favourite supplement is made by Patrick Holford. It's called Connect, and it combines all the necessary vitamins in one capsule.

Tests

See Resources for where to buy a homocysteine home test kit.

The more signs and symptoms that apply to you, the higher the chance that you have raised homocysteine levels. But the only way to know for sure is to take a blood test. Urine tests are not as reliable. I make no apologies if your test comes back OK and you feel as if you've wasted your money! Everyone should be checking their homocysteine every five to ten years. The older you are, the more important it is for you to keep your homocysteine levels low.

You're looking for a reading of 6 μmol/L or below. A homocysteine level above 11 leads to brain shrinkage, which is probably why high homocysteine levels are indicated in Alzheimer's (Braly & Holford 2003). And I imagine that brain shrinkage probably causes other unpleasant brain symptoms too.

Anyone with a family history of heart disease should be regularly testing their homocysteine because high levels damage the lining of the arteries. My partner's family has a history of heart disease and so, when I met him, I asked him to check his homocysteine levels. Sure enough, they were excessively high at 12 μmol/L. It took a year to get them below 6, but this was probably because he kept forgetting to take his supplement! It usually takes around six months to correct.

Interestingly, the NHS says levels of up to 15 are safe; however, it's well documented that the risk of coronary artery disease is high with levels between 10–15 μmol/L. Evidence shows that each increase of 5 μmol/L increases the risk of coronary heart disease by approximately 20 per cent (Humphrey et al 2008)!

Inflammation and brain symptoms

If you have gut dysbiosis, you almost certainly have an inflamed gut. And if you have mental health issues, you may have inflammation in your brain. So, what exactly is chronic inflammation? Simply put, it's the body's defence mechanism. The body identifies incoming toxins and stimulates white blood cells to protect us from infection. The problem is that we're constantly bombarded and so the body's immune response is constantly firing. Subsequently, the body's normally protective immune system eventually causes damage to its own tissues.

Risk factors

There are many things in our modern-day life that can cause inflammation – chemicals from our environment, obesity, stress, insomnia, some prescription drugs – but probably the worst offender is the Western diet because it's full of processed, sugary foods, and excess sugar floating around your bloodstream causes inflammation.

We're bombarded from every angle with toxic, inflammatory factors! You can see how our diet and lifestyle lends itself so beautifully to chronic inflammation and disease. Inflammation is damaging to both physical and mental health.

Interesting titbit

Just one bad meal choice, such as a microwave meal, can cause your rate of inflammation to skyrocket and remain high for several hours. Most Westerners regularly eat high-carbohydrate, processed foods, which is why we're a nation of inflamed people.

Signs and symptoms

Inflammation is associated with a whole range of brain symptoms, from anxiety to OCD. Inflammation activates the release of inflammatory cytokines and immune cells, both of which have been shown to access the brain and alter mood and behaviour. Cytokines also affect neurotransmitters such as serotonin and dopamine. This impacts neurocircuits in the brain, leading to depression and anxiety disorders (Miller et al 2013). The good news is that you can reduce your inflammation and so your brain symptoms should also reduce.

Take a look at the following questions and see how many you answer yes to. If my clients answer yes to three or more, I suspect they have chronic inflammation.

» Do you have the classic symptoms of an inflamed gut – diarrhoea, acid reflux, abdominal pain, blood or mucus in your poop, and other digestive disturbances?
» Do you have depression, anxiety or any other mood disorders?
» Have you been diagnosed with an autoimmune condition?
» Do you get joint and muscle pain?
» Do you suffer from poor sleep or sleep apnoea?
» Do you have skin conditions such as rosacea, psoriasis or rashes?
» Have you had unexplained weight gain or weight loss?
» Do you suffer from fatigue?

Interesting titbit

Did you know that depression is classed as an inflammatory condition? The more depressed you are, the more inflamed you are likely to be (Howren et al 2009). It regularly surprises me that my depressed clients haven't been told this. If you approach depression from the angle of reducing inflammation through diet and supplements, it puts you back in control.

Inflammation and obesity

Inflammation encourages brain symptoms such as impulsive and addictive behaviour (Heber & Carpenter 2011).

This can cause you to crave and binge on rubbish foods. But the more rubbish foods you eat, the more inflamed you'll become. It's a vicious circle! This could explain overeating by obese people. Obesity is associated with inflammation, which may cause addictive behaviours around food. If this sounds like you, you mustn't be critical of yourself because it has nothing to do with willpower or self-control. It's all down to how inflamed you are. I hope it will lift your spirits now that you understand that you're not weak when you make poor food choices. You're simply a victim of your inflammation. So, please be kind to yourself.

I've noticed another behavioural pattern in my binge-eating clients: they often lack self-respect, and binge eating is a sort of punishment or self-harm. If you think this applies to you, it may be worth treating the root cause of your lack of love for yourself before you tackle my three-point plan. Making dietary changes can be tough. If you don't love and respect yourself enough to put in the effort, you may be setting yourself up for failure, which would only perpetuate your feelings of frustration with yourself.

Treatment

Avoid highly inflammatory foods such as sugar, gluten, processed foods and red meat, reduce carbohydrates, moderate your alcohol intake, exercise regularly, get good quality sleep, implement lifestyle changes that will lower stress levels and take supplements such as turmeric, berberine, omega 3 and vitamin C.

All the above are part of my three-point plan, which should help you to lower your inflammation. A healthy diet has been proven to keep inflammation under control. Conversely, an unhealthy diet and lifestyle have been shown to promote inflammation. This is probably one of the reasons why the three-point plan has been so effective in helping my clients because it reduces inflammation.

Cerebral allergy

In this book, I discuss allergies and intolerances to foods and their effects on the digestive system. But allergies and intolerances don't only affect digestion; they can cause all sorts of unpleasant brain symptoms too. Cerebral allergy is another term for brain allergy. Allergies and intolerances are common in people suffering with gut dysbiosis and recent research is linking gut dysbiosis to cerebral allergies. A brain allergy is any overreaction of the immune system to a food or substance that creates emotional, psychological or neurological symptoms (Zhou et al 2019). Patients with a combination of gut and brain symptoms tend to have overstressed, overreactive immune systems, making them more prone to allergies and intolerances. These people often feel mentally calmer when fasting, which can be an indication of cerebral allergies.

Interesting titbit

I once read a fascinating case study about a young woman who had been institutionalised several times after psychotic episodes. She was permanently prescribed strong tranquillisers to keep her calm. Her family continually looked for a cause of her illness, and after removing dairy products from her diet, she made a complete recovery. She was weaned off her medication, went to university and led a normal, fulfilling life. But what wasn't mentioned in this case study was her digestive health. I'd be interested to know if she suffered from gut symptoms. I'd like to bet that she did!

Signs and symptoms

Anxiety, brain fog, confusion, depression, panic attacks, psychosis, phobias.

Risk factors

Cerebral allergies can be caused by chemicals, dust, pollen or by foods. Common triggers are wheat, milk, corn and eggs. The effects of these foods tend to be delayed, making them hard to identify. Gut dysbiosis, pyrrole disorder and cerebral allergy often go hand in hand.

Treatment

Supplements: B3 has an antihistamine effect, which can help cerebral allergy. I also recommend vitamin C, zinc, B6 and manganese.

Tests

If cutting out the recommended foods included in my three-point plan doesn't ease your symptoms, I suggest you take a food intolerance test and also a food and environmental allergy test.

Hormone imbalance

Hormones are your body's chemical messengers and they coordinate many different functions in your body. Some hormones have a direct and profound impact on mental health (Hwang et al 2020). Anyone who has experienced premenstrual tension (PMT) knows that hormones can affect emotions but in some people hormone imbalances can cause severe brain symptoms such as anxiety, depression, paranoia and psychosis.

Signs and symptoms

Anxiety, depression, panic attacks, mood swings, fatigue, sleep issues, reduced sex drive, difficulty having orgasms, vaginal dryness, mood swings, thinning hair, weight gain, loss of bone density.

Risk factors

So, what causes hormone imbalance? A diet high in refined carbohydrates can cause insulin resistance, which negatively impacts hormone balance. Insulin is the master hormone. Eating a diet low in carbohydrates, as laid out in this book, reverses insulin resistance therefore balancing all hormones. Stress is another contributor, as are vitamin and mineral deficiencies. Medications such as statins can also cause disruption. And the chemicals found in our modern-day environment, such as pesticides and plastics, which find their way into our foods and drinking water, are also major disruptors.

Thyroid deficiency is a common hormone imbalance and over the years I've seen it in a lot of my clients. Symptoms include poor concentration, memory problems, panic attacks, indigestion, constipation, dry skin, cold hands and feet, poor temperature control, weight gain and insomnia. A common sign of an underactive thyroid, which I've seen in many of my clients, is thinned and partly missing eyebrows.

I don't believe thyroxin should be prescribed until the patient has tried a more natural approach. We must consider why thyroxin levels are low. Iodine deficiency is epidemic and has been linked to an underactive thyroid and breast cancer. I've taken an iodine supplement for years. Dairy products, being overweight and stress all compete with thyroxin. Tyrosine, selenium, zinc, and iodine all support the thyroid.

Case study

One of my clients, a woman in her late forties, was experiencing depression and exhaustion. Her GP had diagnosed her with chronic fatigue syndrome and recommended bed rest and antidepressants. She consulted me because she wanted to understand the root cause of her malady. She experienced small improvements following my three-point plan but not as great an improvement as most of my clients. I recommended several blood tests, one of which showed she was severely deficient in testosterone. She consulted a private GP who prescribed testosterone therapy and the improvement in her mental and physical health was astounding.

Interesting titbit

Progesterone dampens epinephrine (adrenaline) and the fight-or-flight response. This is why, when progesterone levels fall during the menopause, women often feel anxious (Toriizuka et al 2000). A pattern I've noticed in quite a few of my menopausal clients is that they crave an alcoholic drink on most evenings. Alcohol also dampens epinephrine and the fight-or-flight response, so this could explain their craving.

Treatment

As a basic rule of thumb, a clean diet that's low in sugar, a relaxed lifestyle and a basic vitamin and mineral programme as laid out in my three-point plan may be enough to keep detoxification pathways open and redress a hormone imbalance. It's hard to avoid the chemical onslaught so just do your best; filter your water, eat organic food and use cleaning and personal care products made with natural ingredients.

More research is needed into the link between mental health and hormones to ensure that patients get the correct treatment because if hormones are the root cause of mental health problems, then no amount of psychiatric medication will correct the issue. For this reason, I encourage clients to test their hormone levels before accepting antidepressants or anti-anxiety medication.

Tests

» Thyroid function test.
» Dried Urine Test for Comprehensive Hormones (DUTCH test).
» HbA1c blood sugar test.

Unstable blood sugar levels

Blood sugar levels are the measure of glucose in the blood. The level should ideally be balanced and consistent. If blood sugar levels are continuously fluctuating between high and low, it can cause unpleasant brain symptoms. If you've ever woken up during the night feeling highly anxious, it could be due to a dip in blood sugar levels.

Signs and symptoms

Sweating, tiredness, shaking, palpitations, headache, stomach ache, muscle aches, restless legs, insomnia, dizziness and dumping syndrome (rapid gastric emptying). The brain uses glucose from the blood to function, so fluctuations in blood sugar can cause brain symptoms such as nervousness, crying, anxiety, panic, depression, brain fog, phobias and confusion.

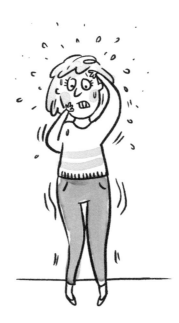

Risk factors

The Western diet is high in refined carbohydrates, which cause blood sugar fluctuations, and so I recommend a diet low in refined carbohydrates, as laid out in this book. Other causes of unstable blood sugar levels are vitamin and mineral deficiencies or prolonged periods of stress. Stress can lead to adrenal exhaustion, which may result in hypoglycaemia (low blood sugar).

Treatment

» My number one supplement for stabilising blood sugar is chromium.

» Glucomannan just before a meal lowers insulin levels.

» One capsule of berberine with each meal helps to keep blood sugar levels stable.

» Blood sugar levels can be particularly unstable after a bad night's sleep, so I recommend a low-carb breakfast such as scrambled egg and avocado on almond bread (see Recipes).

Tests

You can check your blood sugar levels at home on a daily basis using a simple finger-prick blood test. Kits such as Accu-Chek are available to buy online.

Or an HbA1C test (see Resources) can show your average blood sugar levels over the past few months.

Interesting titbit

Metabolic syndrome is a cluster of conditions associated with diabetes, stroke and heart problems. The World Health Organization has cited metabolic syndrome as a highly prevalent disease. One of the signs of metabolic syndrome is high levels of glucose in the brain. Structural brain changes have been seen in people with metabolic syndrome. It causes brain atrophy and the shrinkage of grey matter, the same as people with pre-dementia. I feel sure this must produce some unpleasant brain symptoms which could possibly be misdiagnosed as a mental illness (Kordestani-Moghadam et al 2020).

Metabolic disorders of the brain

Metabolism is the process of turning food into energy. Mental illness can be connected to metabolism or, more specifically, to mitochondrial dysfunction (Gardner & Boles 2011). Mitochondria are the powerhouses of our cells and they regulate metabolism. All the various labels of mental disorders from schizophrenia and depression to anxiety have one pathway in common: metabolism. This is a huge subject and so for the full story along with the supporting science, I recommend you read *Brain Energy* (2022) by Christopher M Palmer, who has worked for 25 years as a psychiatrist and neuroscience researcher. He recognised that many of his patients didn't get better with the current pharmaceutical approach until, one day, he recommended one of his patients with schizophrenia follow a ketogenic diet for weight loss, and the happy by-product of this was a dramatic reduction in his patient's psychiatric symptoms.

This set Palmer on a journey, digging into the medical literature to discover the connection between metabolism, metabolic disorders and mental illness. The ketogenic diet has a profound effect on brain metabolism, and I'll be discussing it more in a later chapter. But there are other things besides following a ketogenic diet that you can do to improve your mitochondrial function: intermittent fasting, eliminating refined foods, eating organic pasture-raised meat, antioxidant supplements and antioxidant-rich foods, exercise, stress reduction, eight hours of quality sleep, cold exposure therapy, berberine and green tea. I recommend all the above as part of my three-point plan and you'll be reading a little about each of them later in the book. Perhaps this is another reason why I get great results from my three-point plan because it improves mitochondrial function.

Blood–brain barrier permeability

I'd like to touch on the blood–brain barrier because it relates to the gut microbiome and mental health. The blood–brain barrier is a very thin membrane surrounding your brain. It acts as a filter, allowing nutrients to cross over into your brain while keeping unwanted toxic molecules out of it. A healthy, properly functioning blood–brain barrier is essential for optimal mental health, but unfortunately it can become damaged and leaky, allowing toxins to enter the brain.

Signs and symptoms

Anxiety, depression, schizophrenia and ADHD.

Risk factors

Several things can cause damage to the blood–brain barrier, including stress, inflammation (Sankowski et al 2015), intestinal permeability (leaky gut syndrome), poor diet such as high fat content and excessive alcohol (Pendyala et al 2012), and environmental toxins. You can see from the above list that the risk factors for both gut dysbiosis and blood–brain barrier damage are the same. Perhaps this explains why gut symptoms and brain symptoms go hand in hand.

> **Interesting titbit**
> Have you heard of glyphosate? It's the most widely used herbicide worldwide. It has been shown to cross the blood–brain barrier and cause inflammation and is another reason why you should eat organic foods wherever possible (Winstone et al 2022).

Treatment

Limit alcohol intake, reduce stress, take omega 3 supplements, get good quality sleep, meditation, rest, detox. The blood–barrier can be healed in much the same way as the gut, so my three-point plan will benefit both.

Tests

There are tests available but they're quite pricey and I've never recommended them to my clients.

Case study

The woman in this case study had several of the conditions we've just looked at and is a classic example of how conditions can overlap. Her main symptoms were alternating constipation and diarrhoea, anxiety and panic attacks. We ran tests to check intestinal function, kryptopyrroles, copper, vitamins and minerals, methylation and oxidative stress. Her stool test showed a deficiency in bifidobacteria, which is a good bacterium; a moderate amount of an entamoeba parasite; a large amount of yeast, cultured as *Candida albicans*; a few strains of bad bacteria, such as strep and low amounts of butyrate (an important fatty acid). From these results plus her gut symptoms I concluded that she had gut dysbiosis.

Her kryptopyrrole test was 6.85, which isn't especially high but high enough to treat for pyrrole disorder. Her copper levels were raised, at 18.73; ideally, they should be at 12 or lower. Zinc levels were adequate at 13.3 but this put the ratio of copper to zinc at 1.4:1, whereas the ideal ratio is 0.8:1. This means her copper levels were way too high compared to zinc. Ceruloplasmin (a protein that binds to and helps excrete copper) was a little low at 0.36. Magnesium levels were in the OK range at 2.15 but benefits are usually felt when they're a little higher. The methylation panel showed she was undermethylating and her homocysteine levels were slightly raised at 8.4. Her glutathione levels were low, suggesting oxidative stress, and she was deficient in vitamin B2.

Treatment plan

My first port of call is always the gut. There's no point trying to correct copper and zinc levels with nutritional supplements if your gut can't absorb them. So, for the first month, we focused on the gut.

» **Point 1: Diet.** My diet recommendations, as laid out later in this book, plus butyrate-rich foods such as coconut oil and walnuts, and foods rich in zinc such as beef, crab, chicken, nuts and seeds.
» **Point 2: Lifestyle.** Daily walks using ankle weights as a way of taking time for herself and losing a few pounds.
» **Point 3: Supplements.** After two weeks of following a clean diet, by which time hopefully her gut would be less inflamed, we introduced an antimicrobial to clear the gut of *Candida* and parasites, betaine HCL to aid digestion and help kill off imbalanced strains of bacteria, and after a month on these supplements a probiotic containing bifidobacteria. I'll explain more about these supplements in a later chapter.

After four weeks of following the above plan, she continued with my recommendations and also introduced zinc picolinate, starting at 30 mg a day and working up very slowly to 90 mg a day. Zinc helps to excrete copper but we didn't want her to excrete it too quickly because it could exacerbate symptoms. Zinc is also essential to help correct pyrrole disorder and aid methylation.

We also added antioxidant drops containing vitamins A, E, D and K because pyrrole disorder causes oxidative stress. Vitamins A and E also help lower copper and increase ceruloplasmin. Then we added a B6 supplement in the form of P5P to decrease pyrroles and copper levels, plus magnesium, colloidal B2 and glutathione. Have you noticed that many of the supplements I've mentioned treat multiple conditions? Not only are the conditions I've mentioned related, but so too are their remedies.

This client had a lot of issues to correct and so recovery was slow but steady. She felt mild relief from her digestive issues within a couple of weeks and from her anxiety within a few months. And things just kept getting better and better. She later followed the ketogenic diet and saw another improvement in her brain symptoms. She felt so well and so calm she went on her first holiday abroad in 27 years! We've yet to retest but the results speak for themselves. She will probably have to stay on a low-dose maintenance programme of supplements and a clean diet for life to feel really well on a long-term basis.

Chapter 5

Conditions related to gut dysbiosis

The following conditions are ones I regularly come across in my practice. If you have gut dysbiosis, you're highly likely to have at least one of the following underlying conditions. This is because everything in the body is connected, so when the gut microbiome is out of kilter, it has a knock-on effect on other bodily systems. All the following conditions are connected to both gut and brain symptoms, and all will be helped by following my three-point plan. I have included them in an overview but I could write another book about each of them!

Candida albicans

Yeast is naturally present in the gut and is kept under control by our friendly internal bacteria. But processed foods, alcohol, stress, antibiotics and the contraceptive pill upset the delicate balance of our internal flora and fauna, causing gut dysbiosis, which allows the yeast to grow and proliferate in a more aggressive form. This is called *Candida albicans*. This form of yeast damages the intestinal barrier, allowing translocation of *Candida* into the bloodstream (Basmaciyan et al 2019). This causes a whole host of symptoms, such as unstable blood sugar levels, psoriasis, eczema, acne, abdominal pain, constipation, diarrhoea, bad breath, food sensitivities, indigestion, gas, painful periods, menstrual irregularities, loss of libido, nasal congestion, watery eyes, ear pain, dizziness, painful joints, vaginal thrush, sore throats, fatigue, mood swings and insomnia.

If your digestive symptoms started after a course of antibiotics, there's a chance you may have *Candida albicans*. *Candida* has been linked to psychiatric problems such as severe anxiety, depression and psychosis. This is caused by the toxic waste products of *Candida* affecting the brain chemistry. Many people, especially women, seem to be affected by this. They can spend years going backwards and forwards to various practitioners looking for an answer, but they're often wrongly labelled as nervy women when, in fact, *Candida* is causing their problem. Women taking oral contraceptives and HRT are at particular risk because oestrogen encourages *Candida* overgrowth. A study from 2016 linked yeast infection to people suffering from bipolar disorder and schizophrenia (Severance et al 2016). The doctors involved in this study urged all clinicians to look for *Candida* infection in patients with mental illness.

Treatment

There's a tried and tested anti-*Candida* protocol you can follow. The treatment has four points:

1. Starve the *Candida* by cutting out of your diet all the foods that feed it. This includes sugar in all its forms, plus yeast, dairy products, refined carbohydrates and alcohol.
2. A supplement programme to boost immunity and detoxify the body.
3. Antifungals to kill the *Candida*.
4. Probiotics to re-establish a healthy gut microbiome and keep *Candida* in check.

As the *Candida* starts to die off, it's normal to feel worse before you feel better. For this reason, I recommend you enlist the support of a nutritionist.

Candida albicans used to be recognised by the medical profession. Doctors would automatically prescribe nystatin, an antifungal medication, alongside every prescription of antibiotics, specifically to prevent the overgrowth of yeasts and fungus and therefore protect the gut microbiome. Nowadays, not only have doctors stopped prescribing nystatin, but some of them deny the existence of *Candida* overgrowth altogether, despite the availability of tests that check for its presence.

Auto brewery syndrome is a bizarre condition related to *Candida albicans*. It's where yeast overgrowth in the gut causes carbohydrates to ferment and produce ethanol (alcohol), causing the person to feel drunk without actually drinking alcohol – it even causes the person to test positive on a breathalyser! Consider the other physical and mental symptoms alcohol causes: headaches, brain fog, fatigue, nausea, anxiety, panic attacks, low mood. You get the picture. Fermenting yeast overgrowth can make you feel terrible!

If you can relate to the symptoms I've mentioned above, you have nothing to lose and everything to gain by following an anti-*Candida* treatment plan. My three-point plan will go a long way towards reducing *Candida* overgrowth.

Leaky gut

Another term for leaky gut is 'intestinal permeability'. This is when the lining of the intestine becomes damaged, allowing undigested foods to leak through the gut wall into the bloodstream. The lining of the gut is made from a single layer of cells, meaning it's very thin. These cells are linked tightly together by junctions. These junctions are usually strict about what they allow to pass through from the gut to the body. But when they become damaged, they can no longer do their job properly and bacteria leaks from the gut into the bloodstream. Once in your system, the bacteria can migrate anywhere! This is called bacterial translocation. If bacteria migrate to the brain, they could cause brain symptoms (Twardowska et al 2022). If they migrate to the urinary tract, they could cause cystitis. This may be the first time you've read this information. It can be quite hard to comprehend that symptoms that seem totally separate from your digestion could be caused by your gut. A study identified that the translocation of gut bacteria may play a direct role in major depression. The authors of the study suggest all patients with major depression should be tested for leaky gut syndrome (Maes et al 2008).

So, what causes a leaky gut? Alcohol, sugar, gluten, grains, processed foods and genetically modified (GM) foods can all irritate the gut lining. Other risk factors include gut dysbiosis, *Candida* overgrowth, weakened immunity, stress, food intolerances, antibiotics, painkillers, non-steroidal anti-inflammatory drugs (NSAIDs) and environmental toxins. Signs that you might have a leaky gut include digestive issues, allergies, fatigue, asthma, eczema, acne, rosacea, autoimmune diseases, joint pain, headaches, migraines, thyroid issues, mood swings, weight gain, brain symptoms, yeast infections and food sensitivities.

How to heal a leaky gut

Remove foods that irritate your gut, reduce stress levels, improve the gut flora and fauna with probiotics, repair the wall of the intestines with vitamins A and D and glutamine (Dos Santos et al 2010), and assist digestion with digestive enzymes. My three-point plan should successfully heal a leaky gut.

Small intestinal bacterial overgrowth (SIBO)

SIBO refers to an excess and imbalance of bacteria in the small intestine. SIBO and gut dysbiosis go hand in hand and affect millions of people who eat a Western diet (Achufusi et al 2020). The overgrowth of bacteria ferments any carbohydrates that you eat rather than digesting them. I like to call it 'brewing upper gut' because the process reminds me of brewing beer! Bacteria are not supposed to live in the upper gut and food is not supposed to ferment in the upper gut. Food is supposed to only ferment lower down, in the large intestine. The small intestine should be a sterile place with no fermentation. Stomach acid keeps it sterile.

What causes SIBO?

A depletion of stomach acid allows SIBO to take hold. Various things can cause stomach acid to deplete: old age, nutritional deficiencies, stress and wrongly prescribed antacid medication. If your digestive symptoms started after taking antacid proton pump inhibitor (PPI) drugs, there's a good chance you have SIBO. The reason PPIs cause SIBO is because stomach acid is needed to keep the stomach sterile, but PPIs wipe out stomach acid, allowing bad bacteria to proliferate (Fujimori 2015).

Symptoms

The obvious symptoms of a brewing upper gut are bloating, burping, breaking wind, constipation, diarrhoea, acid reflux, nausea and tummy ache. One of the common symptoms that clients with SIBO complain about is indigestion. They describe it as a full feeling or a lump low down in the gullet. But the knock-on effects can be far reaching and include allergies, inflammation, chronic fatigue syndrome, headaches, acne, arthritis, brain fog and brain symptoms. SIBO also leads to inadequate digestive enzymes and an inability to absorb vitamins and minerals. B12 deficiency is common in people who have SIBO, and so are low ferritin levels. But even more insidious are the mental health symptoms caused by the toxins and alcohols released from fermenting foods (Kossewska et al 2022).

Treatment

There's a straightforward breath test that can diagnose SIBO, which measures levels of hydrogen or methane gas. High levels indicate that brewing and fermenting are occurring in your upper gut. The overgrowth of microbes in the small intestine feeds on and ferments sugary foods. The dietary recommendations I make as part of my three-point plan are naturally low in refined carbohydrates, which will starve those pesky microbes. Another thing that helps the stomach restore its natural acid balance is fasting. When the stomach is empty, it can cleanse and rebalance itself. So, try to eat all your meals for the day within a six- to eight-hour window. Another helpful tip is not to overeat because it overwhelms your digestive system and will likely result in the food fermenting in your upper gut. Your body is working hard every minute of every day to be well. All it needs is a little helping hand from you.

Supplements

Digestive enzymes and hydrochloric acid (HCl) will help your stomach digest food rather than ferment it. Vitamin C is an extremely powerful antimicrobial. Taken last thing at night on an empty stomach, it kills bacteria and yeast and sterilises the upper gut. Berberine is also a powerful antimicrobial. Probiotics will help to displace unfriendly gut microbes and repopulate the gut with friendly bacteria. See the chapter on supplements for further information.

Food allergies and intolerances

Most people can eat a wide range of foods without any problems. However, up to 20 per cent of the population react badly to certain everyday foods and eating them may cause uncomfortable physical and mental symptoms (Brazier 2024). This figure is much higher in people with gut dysbiosis. These unpleasant reactions, debilitating as they can be, are most likely to be food intolerances rather than true allergies. Food intolerances may cause uncomfortable symptoms, but only true allergies can be life threatening. Being allergic to a food and being intolerant to a food are two different things. If you have digestive problems and/or brain symptoms, you may suffer from intolerances, so read the next section carefully.

Food allergies

A food allergy is an abnormal immune response to food. The body sees some foods as a threat, and the immune system responds by releasing chemicals such as histamine. These chemicals cause the unpleasant symptoms. An allergic reaction usually occurs soon after eating, making the allergen easy to identify. Symptoms can be as severe as anaphylactic shock. Less severe symptoms include wheezing, itching, skin rashes, sweating, vomiting and swelling of the face and lips. Dairy, yeast, wheat, gluten, alcohol, grains, eggs, nuts, yeast, chocolate, oranges, additives, tea, coffee, alcohol and shellfish are all common trigger foods. Thankfully, it's less common for fruit, vegetables and other nutrient-rich foods to cause an allergic reaction. You know what I'm going to say – keep a food journal!

Discovering your allergy triggers

Food allergy testing is the most reliable method. I'd suggest contacting YorkTest (see the Resources). Testing isn't usually necessary, though because food allergies occur so soon after eating that it's easy to figure out which food is the cause. Foods that provoke an allergic reaction usually need to be avoided for life.

Food intolerances

Fortunately, food intolerances, also known as food sensitivities, tend to be less severe than food allergies. However, they're much more common and can affect any organ or tissue, including the gut and the brain. Food intolerance symptoms come on much more slowly than a food allergy and can take up to three days to manifest. This makes it difficult to identify the offending food. Another factor that makes it difficult to pinpoint is that some people are intolerant to several different foods.

Some common offenders are listed below, but be aware that your own personal food intolerance could be something obscure!

» coffee
» tea
» grains
» wheat
» gluten
» dairy
» high-fibre foods

» chocolate
» sugar
» corn
» soya
» yeast
» eggs
» garlic
» oats
» lentils
» chilli
» peanuts.

Signs and symptoms

Physical symptoms can include tummy ache, diarrhoea, bloating, nausea, vomiting, sweating, headache, migraine, stuffy nose, itchy skin, eczema, water retention, arthritis, underactive thyroid, dark circles under the eyes, water retention, fatigue, sore throat and insomnia. Intolerance can also be associated with a history of hay fever, eczema or asthma. A rapid heartbeat is another common symptom. This can cause anxiety and panic if the sufferer worries that something serious is wrong with their heart.

Brain symptoms

Food sensitivities can cause mental health problems such as irritability, nervousness, anxiety, panic attacks, depression, hyperactivity, schizophrenia and aggression (Food for the Brain Foundation 2024).

Testing

An IgG blood test is a great way of discovering which foods you're sensitive to. These are available from YorkTest (see Resources). Record the results in your food and poop journal.

Causes

As with most of the conditions I've mentioned, I think food intolerances often start with gut dysbiosis. A leaky gut can also cause food allergies and intolerances because when undigested food particles leak through the gut wall into the bloodstream, the body identifies them as foreign invaders. Stress is another cause. When we're under stress, our immunity is suppressed and the digestive tract is no longer protected, leading to food sensitivities. Another cause is enzyme deficiency. As we get older, we make fewer digestive enzymes, meaning our food is only being partially digested. The body can't deal with partially digested foods, and this may trigger a food intolerance reaction. Other common suggested causes of food intolerance include nutrient deficiencies, alcohol, not being breastfed, too clean an environment during childhood, a parent with allergies and medications such as antacids, antibiotics and NSAIDs.

Treatment

Because food sensitivities can have multiple causes, it isn't enough just to remove the offending food. Instead, it's important to follow my three-point plan to truly heal your gut and gain long-term relief. As part of my plan, I invite clients to stop eating the common triggers. Unfortunately, the foods we crave are often the foods we are allergic/intolerant to! Not fair, is it? I'm a big believer in intuition when identifying your problem foods, so trust your gut.

Interesting titbit

A healthy gut microbiome is needed to deactivate histamine. This could be one of the reasons why my clients tell me their allergies and hay fever improve after they have corrected their gut dysbiosis.

Parasites

Parasites are all around us – in our food, on our pets. We can pick them up from other people and reinfect ourselves. A parasite is anything that lives on us or in us, feeding off us and excreting its waste inside us. They take up residence in your gut, your major organs and in your brain. They can cause symptoms such as IBS, weight loss, fatigue, nausea, brain symptoms, insomnia and even cancer.

We are in a new era of parasitism based on pollution. Body care products, exhaust fumes, deodorants, medications, pesticides – all of these find their way into our bodies and react with parasites. The most common way to become infected is through undercooked meat. Other causes include contaminated water, contact with contaminated faeces and poor hygiene. They can easily take up residence in a gut weakened by dysbiosis or *Candida*.

Parasites are notoriously difficult to detect through stool samples, and it may take several samples before they're identified. Blood tests are another way of detecting the antibodies your body would produce if you had a parasitic infection. Your doctor can give you medications to treat parasites and it's possible to follow a supplement programme that kills off the parasites invading your body.

Blastocystis hominis is a parasite that causes all the typical IBS symptoms: bloating, diarrhoea, nausea and wind. It also causes multiple food sensitivities (Shafiei et al 2020). If you've tried excluding foods in the past but have found that as quickly as you remove one food, you develop an intolerance to another, it may be worth testing for this pesky little parasite. For the full story on parasites and their detrimental effects on our health, I recommend Hulda Clarke's book *The Cure for All Diseases* (1995). All the herbs she recommends are available online (see Resources).

Adrenal exhaustion

This occurs when the adrenal glands stop functioning properly as the result of long-term stress. The adrenals are located above the kidneys and produce various hormones, including epinephrine (adrenaline) and cortisol, the stress hormone. Symptoms include all-day fatigue with more energy in the evening, difficulty sleeping, food cravings, low immunity, depression, low libido, fat on the abdomen, inability to concentrate, digestive problems and brain symptoms.

Like everything else we've discussed, you might notice that many of these symptoms are relatively generic. When you've been keeping your journal for some time, you'll notice patterns of stress. Look out for mental/emotional stress such as having a sick relative, a stressful job or an unhappy marriage. Then consider physical stress such as overexercising or biochemical stress such as food sensitivities.

The body responds to all these stresses in the same way by releasing cortisol as part of the fight-or-flight response. Cortisol switches off digestion to divert energy to the organs needed to fight or flee. If you're permanently stressed, this process occurs constantly, which eventually exhausts the adrenal glands until they stop functioning correctly. This is when you start experiencing physical symptoms such as exhaustion and the need to rely on stimulants such as coffee to get you through the day. It's usually around this time that digestive problems begin, and it becomes a self-perpetuating problem.

Adrenal fatigue causes gut dysbiosis, and the biochemical stress of dysbiosis causes adrenal fatigue. It becomes a vicious circle. If you suspect you have adrenal exhaustion, it would probably be worth consulting a nutritional therapist who can order a saliva home test kit to diagnose adrenal fatigue and then guide you through a specific treatment protocol (Wilson 2014). But for now, the three-point plan will go a long way to making you feel better because it removes many of the stressors mentioned above. For the full story on adrenal exhaustion, I recommend the book *Adrenal Fatigue* by James L Wilson (2001).

Summing up

Have you noticed a pattern emerging from everything we've discussed so far? It's like a domino effect, where the fall of one system leads to another system's collapse – and it all starts with gut dysbiosis. This leads to *Candida* overgrowth, which leads to leaky gut, which leads to inflammation, which leads to vitamin deficiencies, which leads to pyrrole disorder and copper overload, and so on. Throw in a stressful life event and your already weakened body is likely to develop a mental illness, an autoimmune condition or some other disease. I know I've said it before, but disease really does begin in the gut. And somewhere in the middle of the domino effect, you're likely to receive a diagnosis of irritable bowel syndrome, depression or anxiety – or all of the above! It may feel as if you have endless problems to fix, but actually you don't because all of these conditions and their remedies are related – everything dovetails.

If you're experiencing gut and brain symptoms, you can presume that you're somewhere along the pathway of dominoes leading from gut dysbiosis. You may not have every single one of the conditions I've mentioned, but you're likely to have two or three. But the good news is, whichever conditions you have, the diet and supplement protocol is always similar. Eat clean, nutritious food. Take supplements that heal your gut, replenish your gut microbiome and correct nutritional deficiencies. And learn to manage your stress. It's a simple yet effective, tried and tested formula made up of only three points:

» dietary changes
» lifestyle changes
» nutritional supplements.

Each point will need tweaking slightly to make it specific for your condition(s), but the principle is the same. This should be of some comfort to you, that no matter what your ailment, the path to health is similar. This isn't some whimsical, fanciful notion – good health really can be that simple. I've seen it many times in my clients and in myself – when you nurture yourself, miracles happen.

My favourite tests

Mental illness is only the tip of the iceberg. There are lots of possible biological causes, which you are now aware of. And the good news is, they can all be tested for.

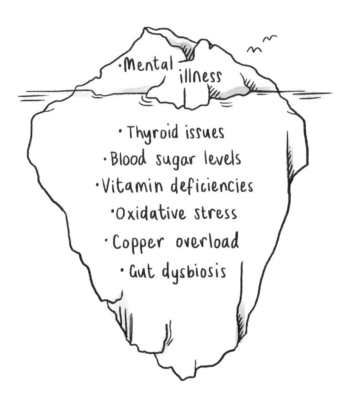

Here's a list of my favourite tests, which will give you a clearer picture of what's going on with your health. You may have to pay privately if you decide you want to go down this road. See Resources at the back of the book for details about where to order tests.

» Kryptopyrrole urine test for pyrrole disorder – available through a private doctor or nutritionist.
» Homocysteine test – this is a finger prick blood test you can do

yourself at home. If homocysteine levels are excessively high, it shows you're not methylating efficiently and you can presume you're deficient in B2, B6, folic acid, B12 and zinc because all these nutrients play an essential role (available online).

» Thyroid panel – possibly available at no cost through your GP.

» Vitamin and mineral testing – available through a private doctor.

» Hair mineral analysis – gives an indication of copper overload and zinc deficiency, also looks at your mineral status and toxic overload (available online).

» Food allergy and intolerance test – finger prick blood test; doesn't need a doctor's referral (order online and do at home).

» HbA1c – from what I've seen in my clients, I believe insulin resistance is rife and can be a cause of brain symptoms; it's also a predictor of all the major diseases, so this is one of my favourite tests. This is a finger prick blood test you can do yourself at home (available online).

» A comprehensive stool test to explore the connection between imbalances in the gut microbiome, absorption of nutrients and mental health. I advise you to do this test with the support of a nutritionist.

» Blood test of serum copper, plasma zinc, vitamin D, magnesium and ceruplasm to check for copper overload and deficiencies (needs a doctor's referral).

I rarely recommend a comprehensive stool analysis to my clients because I find that my three-point plan achieves excellent results, so I only start requesting these tests if they don't see a significant improvement in their digestive symptoms. This means we need to dig a little deeper to discover exactly what's going on. Not all nutritionists would agree with me. Some prefer to know exactly what's going on in the gut before they start recommending dietary changes and supplements. There's no right or wrong way, so if you're working with a nutritionist, just follow their advice.

When it comes to mental health, I take a different approach.

If my clients instinctively feel that their mental health problems are not psychological but have a biological cause, I immediately recommend testing to discover exactly what's gone wrong in the functioning of the body to cause their brain symptoms. A mineral hair analysis to look at zinc and copper levels is one of my favourite tests.

This is an area I feel passionate about. Discovering the cause of an individual's mental health problems is an essential part of recovery. I don't think it's good enough to prescribe antidepressants or counselling without first investigating the cause. Every single one of my clients who consulted me had tried prescription medication and/or counselling with little or no long-term improvement, which led to them feeling neurotic. Tests that reveal a possible physical cause can be extremely reassuring and they empower the sufferer to take control and make practical, life-enhancing changes. An accurate diagnosis is so important. Without this, it's easy to see why you would mistakenly end up on a psychotherapist's couch!

The limitations of testing

Tests such as the hair mineral analysis and vitamin testing are undeniably helpful and are a great indicator of what's going on in your body. But even better is when the test reflects the nutrients' functions in the body. For example, we know that B6 has lots of important functions in the body and low blood levels are an indicator that these functions aren't being carried out, but a better indicator would be a homocysteine test. If your homocysteine levels are excessively high, we know for sure that there isn't sufficient B6 in your system to carry out its function of keeping homocysteine levels low. The best way to determine if a nutrient is functioning in your body is an in-depth symptom analysis alongside your blood tests. When it comes to interpreting a test, a nutritionist will go through an in-depth symptom analysis to see if test results match up with symptoms. This verifies the accuracy of your test results. For this reason, I think it's helpful to work with a nutritionist when interpreting your test results.

Chapter 6

The digestive system

In this chapter, our focus is going to be on digestion. Please don't be tempted to skip this part, however tedious the workings of your gut and the foods you eat may seem! It's all essential information. Digestion is the process of turning the foods you eat into the nutrients your body uses for energy, growth and cell repair. The digestive system takes in nutrients and sends out waste. What you eat, digest and absorb becomes who you are. Healthy digestion is dependent on a healthy gut microbiome. At the risk of sounding like a broken record, good health starts in the gut!

I think it would have been very tricky for me to have recovered from pyrrole disorder and copper overload without also healing my gut. My recovery was dependent on increasing my levels of B6 and zinc, which required my digestive system to be absorbing efficiently. So, I think it's important you understand what's going on.

Bowel habits

Bowel habits vary from person to person. Sudden changes are often harmless, but they can indicate that all is not well with your gut. Monitoring your bowel habits and the consistency of your poop helps you to gauge the health of your gut microbiome. You will soon start to see what is normal for you. Consider the following:

Is your poop consistent in the way it appears? Monitor any changes in the smell, firmness, frequency or colour as it can indicate there's a problem.

» The colour should be medium brown.
» Extremely smelly poop and wind can be an indicator of gut dysbiosis.
» A healthy bowel movement should be painless and require minimal strain.
» Mucus in your poop can be a sign of an inflamed gut.
» It's ideal to go two or three times a day.
» Take time to notice exactly what you're expelling. Yucky, but essential!

Pooping

There are a few important things you should know about passing a healthy bowel movement. One of the most important is that sitting on a toilet is a completely unnatural way for humans to defecate! It goes against our evolutionary development. How do you suppose our ancestors pooped? Let me tell you, they squatted! Now, I appreciate that sitting on a toilet feels much more comfortable and civilised, but it puts us in the wrong position for a complete emptying of our bowels. Squatting encourages the pelvic floor muscles to relax and reduces the need to strain.

I recommend putting a little footstool in your bathroom that you can pop under your feet as you sit on the toilet. Never strain too hard because this can permanently damage the muscles inside your bottom, making it even harder to pass a motion.

Another tip for regulating bowel movements is to eat your main meals at a similar time each day. This helps your gut establish a steady rhythm. People who work shifts are often constipated because their meal and sleep times are constantly changing.

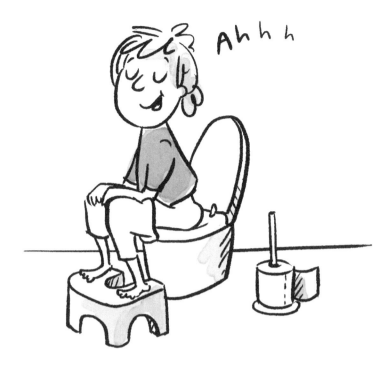

Constipation

This is a major symptom of gut dysbiosis. This is probably because plenty of good bacteria are needed to form a healthy poop but people with gut dysbiosis tend to have more bad bacteria than good. Constipation happens when you don't poop very often, when your poop feels solid and uncomfortable to pass, or you pass a motion regularly but only in tiny amounts. For example, a healthy person generally poops two or three times a day, but some people only go two or three times a week. Just imagine all that old, impacted faeces loitering inside your gut!

When you're constipated and faeces are hanging around in the bowel, autotoxicity can occur. This is when toxins aren't being expelled in your poop, so they are reabsorbed into the bloodstream and travel around your body like dirty dishwater. This can cause unpleasant symptoms such as headache, fatigue and brain symptoms (Mathias 2018).

Symptoms of constipation can vary from person to person. The most common are tummy ache, bloating, hard poop, not going to the toilet every day, tiredness, headache and diarrhoea – yes, diarrhoea! It sounds contradictory, doesn't it? Sometimes when the bowel gets so impacted with faeces, it forces it all out by going into spasms, which cause tummy cramps and diarrhoea. These blowouts are usually quite severe. The cramping can be extremely uncomfortable and you may be sitting on the toilet for some time. Don't worry too much if you think this sounds like you and you're trying to work out whether you should be following a treatment protocol for constipation or for diarrhoea. The remedy is similar for both. It's all about regulating bowel movements and peristalsis (the muscle contractions which push poop through your intestines).

Fibre is great for regulating peristalsis, but it's important to find the right fibre for you because some will worsen your symptoms. Two sources of fibre commonly recommended by doctors are bran and Fybogel, but a lot of my clients have told me these irritate their gut. Ground linseeds are a gentle and effective source of fibre. They are insoluble, which means they don't ferment and cause bloating and wind like some other sources of fibre do. So, if you're a particularly windy person, you'll probably fare well on linseeds. I recommend sprinkling a tablespoon over a meal (they're tasteless). Start off by doing this once a day and build up the amount slowly to your desired dosage. Another great source of gentle fibre is glucomannan. This is from the roots of the konjac plant, and I'll be discussing it in more detail in the chapter on supplements.

Please avoid taking laxatives and stick to natural fibres instead because over time laxatives can make the bowel lazy (Watson 2020), which ironically causes constipation!

Why not test the transit time of your poop? It's simple to do.

1. Don't eat sweetcorn for a week.
2. After a week, eat a generous serving of sweetcorn.
3. Wait for the sweetcorn to reappear!

Inspect each bowel movement for sweetcorn. Ideally, you'll spot the sweetcorn in your poop 24 hours after eating. More than 48 hours indicates that you're constipated.

Causes

The most common causes of constipation are poor diet, not drinking enough water, stress, lack of exercise, some medications, menopause, a change in routine such as holidays or shift work, holding on to negative emotions and regularly ignoring the urge to poop. I've lost count of the number of women (and, in my experience, it's always women) who have told me they'll only poop in their own toilet, in their own home. I can't tell you how damaging this is. Over time it dulls the reflex that tells you when you need to go. If this is a problem for you, please do whatever it takes to overcome it. I'd suggest counselling or hypnotherapy. Try anything – just don't hold on to your poop!

The diet recommendations laid out in this book will help you regulate your bowel movements. But for now, just be aware of what you've been eating. Sugary and processed foods are constipating whereas vegetables, salad, seeds and berries are a great source of gentle fibre. It's important to gain control of constipation because, over time, it may cause piles, diverticulitis and cancer. Colon cancer is one of the nation's biggest killers, so it's worth understanding what causes it and what you can do to prevent it.

Case study

One of my clients came to see me because constipation was getting her down. She only went to the toilet once or twice a week, and laxatives seemed to have stopped working for her. She was developing more and more digestive symptoms (bloating, headaches, nausea), and regularly had such severe stomach cramps that they would keep her awake at night. I asked her to fill in a food and poop journal, and when I saw what she ate, there was no wonder she rarely went to the toilet. Her diet was terrible – basically just processed junk foods and no fibrous, natural, whole foods. I'm surprised she pooped at all!

On a typical day, she ate Coco Pops for breakfast, a white bread sandwich and crisps for lunch, a ready meal for dinner, and she snacked on *lots* of chocolate! Chocolate has been shown to be constipating (Müller-Lissner et al 2005). I know it's hard to believe that anything that tastes as good as chocolate can be bad for you, but sadly it is. She also drank nothing but tea, which is dehydrating and worsened her constipation. Tea has a diuretic effect, meaning it expels water from the body. One can presume that the intestines of a constipated person are pretty dehydrated as it is, so a diuretic is the last thing that's needed. Sadly, the diet I've just described is standard for a lot of people.

And so I implemented the three-point plan. It would be unrealistic to recommend a super-duper healthy diet when someone's diet is as bad as this lady's was because she wouldn't stick to it for long – so I just tweaked her diet slightly. I substituted Coco Pops for porridge, with a sprinkle of ground linseeds. At lunch, she replaced white bread with wholegrain. In the evenings, she would boil some frozen veg to eat alongside her microwave meal. During the day, she would snack on fruit as well as chocolate. I couldn't convince her to drink plain water, but she agreed to drink two pints daily, with a drop of orange cordial added. I also recommended a supplement called Lepicol, which is made up of psyllium husks and probiotics, which add bulk to your faeces and regulate peristalsis. Her bowel had become sluggish and lazy from taking laxatives, so Lepicol was essential to re-educate her bowel. I also recommended she start walking to work as often as possible because exercise massages the bowel and aids peristalsis. So, as you can see, she didn't do anything too drastic. Of course, her diet could still have been better – but it was enough to reduce her symptoms and help her to poop around six or seven times a week.

An interesting thing I've noticed in my clients is that the ones suffering from gut symptoms are generally not as motivated as those who suffer from brain symptoms. As a result, I have to give them a rather tame, watered-down version of my three-point plan. In contrast, my clients with brain symptoms embrace my three-point plan wholeheartedly and are prepared to make big changes for the sake of their mental health.

Diarrhoea

This is frequent, loose, watery poop, usually accompanied by gut cramps and spasms. Diarrhoea is a common symptom of gut dysbiosis. I think it's helpful if you can identify what's causing your diarrhoea, so I encourage my clients to look for correlations in their food, mood and poop journal. I've noticed that a lot of my clients see an improvement when they remove gluten, dairy and sugary foods from their diet and lower their stress levels. In my experience, these are the main triggers but be aware that your personal trigger could be something different. The majority of my clients see an improvement in symptoms when following my three-point plan.

Some other common causes are caffeine, alcohol, food intolerances, constipation, a lack of digestive enzymes, the side effects of medication or excessive exercise (Arasaradnam et al 2018). Gentle fibre helps to stop diarrhoea because it regulates peristalsis in the intestines, which then helps to prevent the spasms and cramping that cause diarrhoea. If diarrhoea is a recurring problem for you, it's essential to drink lots of water.

Diarrhoea can be a sign of inflammation. If it's a chronic problem and you have blood or mucus in your poop, it would be worth requesting a colonoscopy, which would show if you have inflammatory bowel disease.

Flatulence

Everyone trumps! But people with gut dysbiosis trump more than others! The amount of wind produced depends on the types of bacteria in the gut microbiome. Some people have a lot of bad gut bacteria, which causes food to ferment, which in turn produces excessive wind. People with a healthy gut full of good bacteria digest their food efficiently and trump much less than those who suffer from digestive troubles.

It's important not to hold in your wind because it can cause crippling tummy ache. One of my clients was married to a chap who disapproved of trumping (I'm sure this should be grounds for divorce!), the result being that she became so severely bloated and constipated that she was hospitalised due to chronic pain. I feel confident that any bloating and wind will decrease as you follow my three-point plan.

Chapter 7

Things that affect gut health

Detoxification

The liver, kidneys, lungs, digestive system, lymphatic system and skin are all part of your body's detoxification system. Detoxing is an essential bodily function that's constantly taking place. It's how the body rids itself of potentially harmful substances. Unfortunately, we regularly take in more toxins than the body can handle. Most toxins we ingest are via poor food choices such as processed foods, additives, sugar, coffee and alcohol. Other sources of toxins include smoking, medication, pollution, body care products, exhaust fumes, pesticides and household cleaning products such as washing-up liquid and furniture polish.

There are also other factors that put added pressure on your detoxification system, such as a lack of sleep, stress and nutritional deficiencies. Another common cause of toxic overload is gut dysbiosis because one of the ways the body expels toxins is in our poop. So, it's important to help your body to detox.

Imagine you're cleaning a filthy house, and while you're cleaning, someone is throwing in more rubbish – but they're throwing it in quicker than you can clean it up. So, what do you do? You start to hide some of the mess in cupboards and drawers and plan to deal with it at a later date. This is precisely what your body is constantly doing. It strives to keep on top of all the bad foods and toxins, but when it's overwhelmed, it stores the toxins in your fatty tissue. For this reason, some people who struggle to lose weight find that weight drops off easily when they detox because it allows the body to process the toxins it has stored (Jackson et al 2017).

If you relate to five or more of these symptoms, you'll likely need to detox:

» irritable bowel syndrome
» excessive mucus
» strong body odour
» nausea and sickness
» low alcohol tolerance
» mood swings
» poor immunity, regular colds and infections
» food sensitivities
» joint aches and pains
» dark-coloured urine
» feeling run down
» skin problems such as acne, eczema, psoriasis
» low energy and always tired
» frequent headaches
» cellulite
» watery, itchy, red or swollen eyes
» dark circles under the eyes
» brain symptoms such as anxiety, depression and panic.

There have been scientific studies proving that exposure to and accumulation of toxins plays a significant role in cardiovascular disease, type 2 diabetes, obesity and cancer (Hodges & Minich 2015). The aluminium found in cancerous breast tissue is an example of toxic exposure from deodorants (Linhart et al 2017).

There are two things we know for sure about detoxing. First, the body has a detoxification system, meaning that detoxing is something the body needs to do; and second, we're exposed to more toxins than previous generations. The conclusion I have come to is that lowering your exposure to toxic substances must be a good thing – but I'll let you draw your own conclusions.

The more I read about the beneficial effects of detoxing and the more I witness its beneficial effects in myself and my clients, the more I champion it and recommend it as a focus to all my clients.

The three-point plan laid out in this book removes many of the more toxic foods and also supports the body's detoxification system. But if you're tempted to do a specific detox, I can recommend the 15-day GI and Liver Detox in Mindy Pelz's book, *The Reset Factor* (2015). By the end of the 15 days, I always have lots more energy.

Interesting titbit

Epsom salt baths are an excellent way to aid detoxification. They contain magnesium and sulphur, both of which help you to detoxify. Simply pour a cupful into your bath and soak for ten minutes.

Fasting

This means abstaining from food and only consuming liquid. It's a great way to detox! Drinking fresh vegetable juices during a fast aids the detoxification process because some plant foods carry toxins out of the body (Mustafe 2021). Fasting has many health benefits: it cleanses your system of old, impacted faeces; it gives the gut a rest; it turns on the body's repair process, known as autophagy; it increases longevity; it improves blood sugar control; it lowers cholesterol and blood pressure; and it reduces inflammation and improves mood (Fond et al 2013).

I use intermittent fasting: I eat my food for the day in a six- to eight-hour window and fast for the remaining 16 to 18 hours. I recommend my clients do the same. So, for example, you could eat your last meal at 6 pm and not break your fast until 10 am the following day. This way, you sleep through the majority of your fast.

We're designed to fast. Our hunter-gatherer ancestors will have had short periods with little or no food. They will also have had extended periods where their diet was purely fruits and vegetables with no meat until their next kill. We're designed by evolution to have periods of feasting, periods of fasting and periods of eating only plant foods, which could be classed as a period of detoxing. Some of my clients have found their mental health symptoms dramatically improve on fasting days. This is an indicator that their brain symptoms could have a biological cause such as food sensitivities.

However, fasting doesn't suit everybody. Some of my clients have told me it can exacerbate their digestive symptoms and some people feel so weak that it's impossible for them to carry on with their daily lives. So don't be disappointed if fasting doesn't suit you. The most important thing is to listen to your body.

Fasting isn't an essential part of my three-point plan. It's optional – but I just want you to be aware of the potential health benefits.

It's important for women to fast in line with their menstrual cycle. The first two weeks of the cycle are the ideal time to do a long fast of 24 hours or more. The last two weeks of the cycle should be focused on eating enough complex carbohydrates to fuel progesterone levels, so fasting shouldn't exceed 18 hours. For the full story, read Mindy Pelz's book, *Fast Like a Girl* (2022).

Absorption

Your intestinal villi play an important part in absorption. The villi are finger-like projections on the small intestine wall which increase the surface area of the small intestine, and this helps you absorb more nutrients. However, gut dysbiosis can damage the villi, which hinders absorption (Ensari 2014). Efficient absorption is an essential part of your recovery, and this is why you *must* correct gut dysbiosis so that you can absorb the vitamins and minerals in your food and supplements. The three-point plan will heal the gut, thereby improving absorption and correcting vitamin deficiencies.

The majority of my clients who pay privately for blood tests are vitamin and mineral deficient, and I believe this is because every one of them is displaying classic symptoms of gut dysbiosis, which prevents them absorbing all the nutrients from their food. We've looked at the consequences that vitamin deficiencies can have on mental health, and this is why I think it's so important to correct gut dysbiosis and absorption issues.

Stomach acid

Hydrochloric acid, also known as stomach acid, is essential for digestion, vitamin and mineral absorption, keeping the stomach sterile and defending against infections. Problems with stomach acid are common, and antacids are big business. But this can be a touchy subject – I believe there's a generation of people that have been wrongly diagnosed as having too much stomach acid when in fact they have too little (Kines & Krupczak 2016)! Many of these people have been wrongly prescribed proton pump inhibitors (PPIs), which have unpleasant side effects and are difficult to stop taking. So, how have we ended up with this misdiagnosis? I think it could be because the symptoms of indigestion (heartburn, lump in throat, cough, bad taste in mouth) all conjure up an image of excess acid. In fact, reflux is typically caused by a *deficiency* of stomach acid. You may be scratching your head and asking yourself, how is this possible? So let me explain the workings of your stomach.

Food travels down your throat and through a sphincter valve into your stomach. This valve is pH sensitive and only closes when there's sufficient acid present in the stomach. The valve is supposed to ensure one-way traffic and keep your food and stomach acid where it belongs, in your stomach. But when there's too little stomach acid, this sphincter flaps open, allowing gastric juices to escape back into the oesophagus, causing all the symptoms I mentioned above. But until levels of stomach acid are raised, the oesophageal sphincter can't function properly.

The best way to increase stomach acid levels is to correct gut dysbiosis and nutritional deficiencies. My three-point plan will show you how to do this by following a clean, nutrient-dense diet and supplementing with probiotics, digestive enzymes and HCl. Research has shown that a clean diet is as effective as PPIs for treating reflux (Herdiana 2023).

Another tip I give my clients is to mix a tablespoon of apple cider vinegar in warm water with a splash of fresh lemon first thing in the morning and before a meal to help raise stomach acid levels and aid digestion.

So, what causes the decline in stomach acid? The symptoms associated with reflux tend to increase with age, while stomach acid production naturally declines with age. Another cause is deficiencies. B vitamins and zinc play an essential role in stomach acid production, and magnesium is needed to support the sphincter valve. But deficiencies in these essential nutrients are common in my practice.

The official name for low stomach acid is hypochlorhydria. Symptoms include: reflux, indigestion, heartburn, upset stomach, nausea, tummy cramps, burping, food allergies, nausea, itching rectum, undigested food in poop, weak, peeling fingernails, dilated blood vessels in cheeks and nose, acne, iron deficiency, paleness and fatigue. The symptoms are similar to having too much stomach acid, so it's easy to get confused!

Diagnosis and home testing

A simple test you can do at home is to take half a teaspoon of bicarbonate of soda mixed in warm water first thing in the morning on an empty stomach. If you have sufficient stomach acid, then the bicarbonate of soda will react with it and make you do several burps. If you haven't burped within three minutes, you probably have hypochlorhydria (low stomach acid)

Proton pump inhibitors

PPIs often cause hypochlorhydria. They strip what little stomach acid you have, meaning your sphincter can't close and your food can't be digested. PPIs will never cure the root cause of your symptoms, and this creates a dependency, despite there being a warning on the label advising they only be taken for four weeks at a time (Ariel & Cooke 2019). If possible, please avoid taking PPIs because they only exacerbate the problem. They actually shut down stomach acid production - destroying your body's ability to produce it! Considering all the things that stomach acid is essential for, I believe this is utter madness. We already know it's needed to close the valve between your stomach and throat. It's also essential to digest your food. It kills harmful bacteria and viruses that enter your system. It helps liberate vitamins, including B12 from your food. As an interesting aside, B12 deficiency is a common side effect of taking PPIs and has been linked to Alzheimer's and dementia (Makunts et al 2019).

So, taking into account all the wonderful things stomach acid does, I have come to the conclusion that ample amounts of stomach acid are a good thing and will give you super-duper digestion! However, please don't suddenly stop taking PPIs, because the rebound effects will be horrible. Follow my three-point plan and withdraw your medication very, very slowly under the guidance of your GP. For occasional reflux symptoms, try natural remedies such as aloe vera juice, baking powder, glutamine or bitters.

Interesting titbit

When my clients present symptoms of gut dysbiosis, I ask them to exclude dairy products as part of the recommendations in my three-point plan. Despite my reassurances, this recommendation almost always triggers concerns about calcium deficiency and osteoporosis. I would estimate that at least half of these people with concerns about osteoporosis had been taking PPIs long term. But *none of them* were aware that PPIs can inhibit the absorption of calcium, leading to reductions in bone mineral density and a high incidence of bone fractures (Khalili et al 2012).

Digestive enzymes

Your body secretes digestive enzymes every time you eat. They are essential to breaking down and digesting your food. If your body doesn't make enough of them, you can't digest food very well, and that can lead to gut dysbiosis, nutritional deficiencies, inflammation, stomach aches, food intolerances, diarrhoea, indigestion, bloating and wind.

Age affects enzyme production, and so the over-fifties may notice they're not digesting their food as well as they used to. This could explain why indigestion often gets worse with age. Vitamin deficiencies can also hinder enzyme production, and many people with gut dysbiosis are deficient due to their digestion and absorption issues. If indigestion is a common problem for you, I suggest trying a digestive enzyme supplement. If you have problems with low stomach acid, look for one that also contains betaine hydrochloride. See the chapter on supplements for recommendations. Digestive enzymes are available in abundance in raw fruits and vegetables. Cooking destroys the enzymes naturally present in food, so don't overcook things. Eating a mix of raw and cooked foods in each meal helps to keep the digestive enzyme content high.

Mucus

In small amounts, mucus is normal and necessary and forms a protective barrier on the surface of the intestines (Paone & Cani 2020). But excessive mucus in your poop is a sign of an unhappy bowel. This often occurs as a result of a poor diet, gut dysbiosis, food intolerances and a chronically inflamed bowel. Sugary foods, wheat, white rice and dairy are all mucus-forming foods. As a child, did you ever make glue from water and flour? Well, if you have a diet high in refined and processed foods, that sticky mess is very similar to the contents of your bowel. The bad bacteria in your gut love mucus – it's a breeding ground for the bad guys! This leads to a downward spiral of gut dysbiosis and inflammation. The three-point plan will naturally clean your bowel and restore good health and function, which should return mucus production to normal levels.

Chapter 8

Food groups

Food and the effect it has on mental and physical health is a huge subject, and one that fascinates me – but I've tried to be as succinct as possible to avoid overloading you with information. We'll look at different food types, and I'll discuss various foods and drinks that I think you should avoid or minimise and why. Then, I'll bring all the information together in the recipe section, which puts all the food information into practical terms with lots of delicious and nutritious meals.

A 2017 study published in *The Lancet* concluded that 'a suboptimal diet is responsible for more deaths than any other risks globally, including tobacco smoking' (GBD 2019). Diet and nutrition play a significant and important role in the overall health of an individual. This is because the food that you eat affects every aspect of your body and mind.

Many people assume that because a food is sold in a supermarket or is commonly consumed it must be healthy and safe. This is not always the case. The food industry is a business and they're more interested in profit than your health. Did you know that the food industry is self-regulated, which basically means it's not regulated (Sharma et al 2010)?!

In order to reduce your gut and brain symptoms and help you live a long, disease-free life, I believe it's necessary to eat a clean and healthy diet. Let's start with the food basics.

Carbohydrates

These are the sugars, starches and fibres found in fruit, vegetables, grains and dairy products. Complex carbohydrates are made by Mother Nature and are found mostly in whole plant foods. Examples include quinoa, sweet potato, asparagus, strawberries, apples and linseeds. These foods are a great source of fibre. Whereas refined carbohydrates tend to be human-made. They are artificial and include foods such as white bread and sugary snacks. These are particularly bad for people with gut dysbiosis. They feed bad gut bacteria and cause gut inflammation, constipation and imbalanced blood sugar levels.

Carbohydrates are made up of different sugars, all varying in size. Glucose and fructose are the two smallest sugars, so they don't require much digesting. These are found mainly in ripe fruit and vegetables. I think they should be the primary carbohydrate source for anyone with gut and brain symptoms.

The next category of carbohydrates is double sugars. Because they're bigger, they're harder to digest. The most common double sugars are lactose, the sugar found in dairy products; maltose, found in starchy foods such as grains; and common table sugar found in confectionery. People with gut dysbiosis can't always break down double sugars. This means they can't be absorbed, so they loiter in the gut and become food for fungi such as *Candida*. This produces toxins that damage the gut wall and negatively affect the body and brain (Campbell-McBride 2004).

Protein

Proteins are commonly found in animal products such as meat, fish and eggs. People with an imbalanced gut microbiome may struggle to digest proteins, resulting in indigestion and tummy ache. If this sounds like you, the digestive enzymes I recommend in the supplement chapter should help. In the meantime, eat plenty of easy-to-digest proteins such as eggs and fish. Also, meats that have been boiled, poached or stewed are easier to digest than those that have been fried or roasted.

Fats

Not all fats are made equal. Some are bad for you and some are extremely good for you. The good fats are called essential fatty acids, so called because they're essential for the correct functioning of the body. Fats that occur naturally in foods such as avocados, eggs, fatty fish, nuts, seeds, cold-pressed olive oil and coconut are all good for your heart health and cholesterol. The fats that are bad for you are trans fats found in processed foods. Also, vegetable and seed oils such as canola oil, sunflower oil, soybean oil, sesame oil and rice bran oil. These are all best avoided as much as possible because too much omega 6 is linked to inflammation and many of the major diseases (Patterson et al 2012).

Fibre

One person's meat is another's poison, and never was this truer than in the case of fibre. For some people, a diet high in fibre is beneficial because it regulates bowel movements, improving both constipation and diarrhoea. But for others, it can irritate digestion. The reason that people's reactions vary is because having plenty of good gut bacteria is essential to digest fibrous foods and not everyone has a healthy balance. This means fibre may sit in the gut for a long time, unable to be digested. This causes fermentation, gas bloating, inflammation and other symptoms typical of gut dysbiosis (Campbell-McBride 2004). So, it's essential to find the right source of fibre for you. Low-sugar fruits, salads, vegetables, linseeds and glucomannan are my preferred sources of fibre. It may be a case of trial and error to discover which sources of fibre your gut can tolerate. Some of my clients have to go easy on fibrous foods until they have improved the diversity of their gut microbiome.

Water

Until the late 19th century, water was a source of illness and contamination. Cholera, dysentery and typhoid were almost always transmitted through drinking water. Around this time, it was discovered that adding chlorine to water killed germs and stopped the spread of disease. Unfortunately, since then, even more chemicals have been added to drinking water, plus other contaminants that find their way into our water supply, such as:

» fluoride
» aluminium sulphate
» calcium hydroxide
» trihalomethanes
» arsenic
» radium
» copper
» lead
» mercury
» pesticides
» hormones
» nitrates
» heavy metals
» antibiotic

... to name but a few!

It seems kind of crazy that the process of making water safe to drink involves adding a load of poisonous chemicals to it, but it doesn't take a genius to work out that this amount of chemical exposure can cause disease. Let me give you a few examples. In areas where there are high levels of fluoride in drinking water, there's a higher incidence of thyroid problems in the community (Peckham et al 2015).

Another disturbing statistic is the link between colorectal cancers and chlorinated water (El-Tawil 2016). Two thirds of our chlorine exposure can come through showering and bathing.

Inhalation of steam and absorption through the skin are just as damaging as drinking, as are chlorinated swimming pools.

Fluoride is routinely added to drinking water in the UK despite it being banned in many other European countries. Fluoride is also found in toothpaste and other dental products. It's known for protecting against tooth decay, but this can so easily be avoided by reducing your consumption of processed sugar. So, if you have a good diet, there should be no need for fluoride. Fluoride is toxic and has been linked to various diseases (Peckham & Awofeso 2014).

An article in the *Guardian* newspaper in March 2023 reported how UK ministers were under pressure to tighten laws on 'forever chemicals' in drinking water. Research shows that people in the UK are subjected to levels that are banned in the US and Europe (Hosea & Salvidge 2023).

The number one concern for people with gut dysbiosis is the effect these chemicals are having on their gut microbiome. You can bet that a dosage of chemicals high enough to kill off deadly bacterial disease is also damaging your gut bacteria. To aid your recovery, you must avoid things that damage the gut microbiome, so I recommend filtering your water.

It's very simple and inexpensive to purify your household water and make it safe for drinking and bathing. There are various water filters on the market. The general rule of thumb is, the more expensive the filter, the more chemicals it removes. For example, reverse osmosis systems are quite pricey, but they remove 99 per cent of chemicals. At the other end of the scale is a Brita or KLAR water filter. Both of these are affordable and still very effective. It's also a good idea to add a shower filter that removes chlorine, pesticides and other chemicals from your bathing water. These are also inexpensive. Ensuring a safe water supply in your home is one of the best investments you can make in your and your family's health.

Drinks

Caffeine is a gut irritant and many people can't tolerate it. A lot of my clients have told me it triggers diarrhoea. I realise it's highly addictive, which can make withdrawal tough, but I urge you to persevere until you master your coffee cravings. As well as being an irritant, caffeine is also a stimulant, and stimulants shut down digestion. So, don't drink coffee at the same time as eating. This also applies to smoking because nicotine is also a stimulant.

Did you know that coffee is *the* most chemically treated food product in the world? Decaffeinated coffee goes through even more chemical processing to remove the caffeine. For this reason, I recommend you only buy organic. This doesn't remove the risks associated with drinking such a chemically contaminated product, but it does reduce them.

Alcohol is another gut irritant. Many alcoholic drinks have a high sugar content, which feeds bad gut bacteria and interferes with the absorption of nutrients. It worsens an already inflamed bowel and contributes to gut permeability. Spirits are particularly harsh.

Processed fruit juices are extremely high in sugar. So, if you fancy a fruit juice, squeeze it yourself and only as an occasional treat. Fizzy drinks and sodas are bad for you, full stop – even the sugar-free ones. I don't feel the need to expand on this – just don't drink them, ever!

Because you're aiming to improve your digestion and overall health, I recommend you drink only filtered water, herbal teas and homemade vegetable juices. I'm a big fan of herbal teas and drink several mugs a day. These are the herbal teas I most commonly recommend to my clients:

» Peppermint tea calms the stomach and reduces bloating. You can use fresh mint from your garden.
» Chamomile tea is calming and relaxing and aids digestion.
» Nettle tea is an excellent liver tonic and stimulates digestion.
» Fennel tea relaxes the stomach muscles to relieve cramping.

Try not to drink too much at mealtimes. When food and liquid enter the stomach together, the liquid dilutes the digestive juices, thus interfering with the digestive process, causing incompletely digested food to move from the stomach into the small intestine. Endeavour to wait 60 minutes after consuming food before drinking large amounts. However, drinking vegetable juice 30 minutes before eating actively aids digestion.

Wheat

Wheat is a predominant ingredient in the Western diet. We find it in bread, pasta, cakes and biscuits, and it's also a 'hidden' ingredient used as a thickening agent in pre-packed sauces, gravy and ready meals. It's a common gut irritant due to the fact that it's highly processed. White flour is no longer a whole grain. It has been over-refined, leaving it nutritionally deficient and harsh on the gut. The wheat we consume today is nothing like the wheat our grandparents would have eaten. This modern strain of wheat is highly addictive. It's also inflammatory and immunoreactive to the gut, brain and nervous system (Scherf 2019). Wheat turns into a gluey mass in our gut. This feeds unhealthy gut bacteria, which produce toxins. These toxins inflame the gut and, in some people, affect brain chemistry and mental health (Ravindran et al 2011).

Did you know it's normal for wheat to be stored for up to two years before food manufacturers purchase it? Two years! Unsurprisingly, it becomes mouldy during this time and enterotoxins grow (Magan et al 2010). These are inflammatory to the gut and brain, and they damage the gut microbiome.

Wheat intolerance has also been linked to schizophrenia. During the Second World War, a now famous study showed a strong correlation between wheat consumption and hospital admissions for schizophrenia. Since then, countless studies have shown a connection between schizophrenia and wheat gluten (Levinta et al 2018). This well-known link has made me wonder what other brain symptoms wheat is causing.

Symptoms of wheat sensitivity include bloating, stomach ache, migraine/headaches, constipation, diarrhoea, depression/anxiety, paranoia, fatigue, acne, sweating, throat troubles and nausea. After reading the above I'm sure you'll understand why wheat is one of the first foods I advise my clients to cut out of their diet. But be prepared for bread cravings!

Label ingredients that can indicate the presence of wheat include: malt, wheat starch, gelatinised starch, hydrolysed vegetable protein, modified food starch, modified starch, natural flavouring, starch, vegetable gum and vegetable starch. Get used to checking ingredient labels when doing your shopping.

Gluten

This is a protein found in some grains, most commonly wheat flour. The name gluten is derived from the Latin word for glue, which tells you something about what it's doing to your insides! Sensitivity to gluten goes as far back as Roman times! Gluten is known to be an intestinal irritant and will provoke some degree of an inflammatory immune response in a high percentage of the population. Coeliac disease and wheat allergy are probably the most well-known conditions related to gluten.

However, there's a whole other spectrum of gluten-related disorders that are generally defined as 'gluten sensitivities' (Sapone et al 2012). These are neither allergic nor autoimmune and therefore not so easy to diagnose as coeliac disease or wheat allergy. Many people spend years going backwards and forwards to their doctor with a wide range of low-level symptoms such as behavioural changes, diarrhoea, nausea, gas, bloating, fatigue, respiratory issues, eczema, osteoporosis, weight loss, depression, thyroid issues, joint pain, nervous system issues, neurological issues, numbness, tingling, balance problems, brain fog, PMS and anxiety. You'll have noticed these symptoms are incredibly diverse.

Gluten sensitivity is hard to diagnose because most labs only test for antibodies to one fraction of the wheat grain. Therefore, traditional blood testing for wheat and gluten intolerance often shows a false negative because the full spectrum of proteins recognised by the immune system aren't tested for. This may lead people to believe their symptoms are psychosomatic, which could be extremely upsetting and confusing. However, these people feel a definite improvement when they exclude gluten from their diet.

So why has gluten become a health problem for so many people? I think part of the problem can be explained by the last section on wheat. Wheat is now a highly toxic, hybridised grain, far removed from its natural state and the strain of wheat gluten eaten by our ancestors (Molberg et al 2005). Plus, we're all consuming more than any other generation, and we're not genetically evolved to digest this amount of gluten. Studies have shown a link between gluten sensitivity and IBS, which makes me think that those with gluten sensitivity have some degree of gut dysbiosis (eg Makharia et al 2015).

Do you remember that we discussed leaky gut syndrome in an earlier chapter and I told you that gluten can be a cause of leaky gut? This is because gluten triggers the release of a protein called zonulin, which controls the junctions between cells in the walls of the intestine. Too much zonulin opens up these junctions, leading to bacterial translocation (Drago et al 2006). High zonulin levels may also be responsible for the breakdown of the blood–brain barrier. This could explain the link between major depressive disorder and increased levels of zonulin.

I think that *everyone* would benefit from eating less gluten. Unfortunately, this is easier said than done because it's such a common ingredient in the Western diet. It's a 'hidden' ingredient in many processed foods such as microwave meals, clarifying agents used in red wine, soups, sauces, emulsifiers, gelling agents, some alcoholic drinks, bread, cakes, pies, cereals, gravy, pasta, salad dressing, soy sauce, ready meals, and some medication and supplements. So, get used to always reading labels! Many ready-made foods labelled 'gluten-free', such as cakes, are highly processed and full of sugar so I recommend that my clients avoid them as much as possible.

Bread has an extremely high gluten content compared to other foods and baking gluten increases its ability to irritate the gut.

Think about your own diet for a moment. How often do you eat bread? How often do you eat other foods containing gluten? Are you consuming gluten on a daily basis? The majority of people do, but it is possible to cut out gluten and still eat a varied and tasty diet.

I realise that changing your diet is daunting and cooking from scratch is time consuming, but the health benefits are worth the effort. Because testing has its limitations, the best way to decide if you're gluten sensitive is to cut out all grains and foods that contain gluten for a few weeks and monitor your symptoms in your food journal. This will give you a pretty good guide as to whether you're reacting to them. I'm confident you won't become nutritionally deficient after cutting out gluten. However, eating gluten may inflame your gut, causing absorption issues that will lead to deficiencies. Gluten sensitivity is not always a lifelong condition, so you may be able to reintroduce it after healing your gut. But I recommend always minimising your intake even if you can eat it without unpleasant effects.

Interesting titbit

In a 2023 interview, Novak Djokovic said that his tennis performance improved dramatically when he cut out gluten! (Gunston 2023)

Grains

Not all grains contain gluten but they all have the potential to be inflammatory to the gut and the brain. Grains, beans, nuts and seeds are designed to *not* be digested! They want to survive digestion in order to be excreted in poop and then replant and proliferate! It's part of their survival mechanism. Because they're hard to digest, they promote gut symptoms. So, for this reason, I usually recommend cutting them all out, at least temporarily while you follow my three-point plan and your gut heals.

If, after a few months, you're feeling better, you could reintroduce small amounts of wild rice, amaranth, quinoa and buckwheat. These are seeds, also known as pseudo grains – they are easier to digest and naturally gluten free. Soaking grains for a few hours before cooking or fermenting them for a week or two before eating also makes them more digestible and less inflammatory to the brain.

If you have brain symptoms be cautious when reintroducing pseudo grains – you may be more susceptible to adverse effects than most people. Although you can't feel an inflamed brain in the same way that you feel when your gut is inflamed, you may still be suffering silently.

For the full story on the detrimental effects grains have on the brain, I recommend David Perlmutter's book, *Grain Brain* (2013). And also, *Gut and Psychology Syndrome* (2004) by Natasha Campbell-McBride. Both are well worth a read.

Dairy products

Dairy intolerance produces an inflammatory response in the body. The severity of symptoms varies but can include excessive mucus production, respiratory problems, asthma, blocked nose and gut symptoms. Lactose is the predominant sugar found in milk and dairy products. Lactose intolerance is the inability to absorb lactose into the digestive system. When it isn't absorbed properly, it can cause abdominal pain, bloating and diarrhoea. Unfortunately, a large percentage of the population struggles with dairy to some degree. This is because our digestive systems have not evolved sufficiently to digest cow's milk. Humans started drinking milk less than 10,000 years ago during the agricultural revolution. I know this sounds like a long time, but it isn't long at all in evolutionary terms. This means milk is not an essential food for adults. We evolved perfectly well without it.

I know this is hard to swallow because we've all been brainwashed to believe milk is essential for us to get enough calcium, but how can this be correct when our evolutionary history proves we developed strong bones without it? No other mammals consume milk beyond their early years. Look at some of the strongest mammals on Earth: lions, tigers, elephants. They don't drink milk beyond infancy, and they certainly don't drink another species' milk like we do! This is because human stomachs are vastly different to a cow's and are therefore unable to properly digest cow's milk.

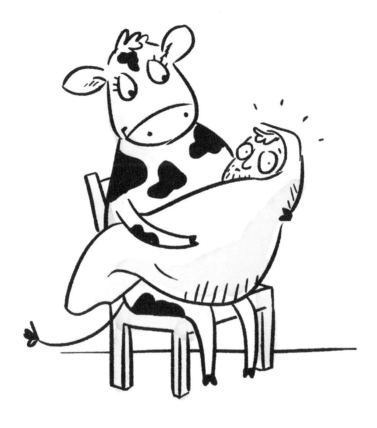

Milk is highly acidic, so to neutralise its effect, the body leeches calcium and magnesium from the bones. So, you see, milk actually *causes* calcium deficiency (iPhysio 2014). Whenever I mention calcium, I also need to mention osteoporosis because my female clients seem to have a morbid fear of it! The World Health Organization has confirmed that countries with low calcium intake don't necessarily have increased cases of osteoporosis. Did you know that osteoporosis is a modern-day disease? Our ancestors, whose diet was similar to the one laid out in this book, didn't get osteoporosis. A diet rich in green leafy veg, seeds and oily fish should be sufficient to safely meet your calcium needs.

For the full story on dairy, I'd recommend reading any of Professor Jane Plant's wonderful books. She dedicated her life to researching the link between diet and cancer. Her scientific studies have shown that dairy is full of added hormones and growth factors, increasing the risk of some cancers. I attended one of her lectures, and she explained the science behind the cancer/dairy link. Let me tell you, it was enough to put me off dairy for life!

The gluten and casein connection

Gluten is the protein found in grains and casein is the protein found in milk. Because they're very similar on a molecular level, they both have similar effects on the body. For this reason, gluten intolerance and casein intolerance often occur together (Ulas et al 2022). Gluteomorphin is an opioid peptide formed during the digestion of gluten, and casomorphin is an opioid peptide formed during the digestion of milk. Perhaps you've heard of opioids such as morphine, opium and heroin? Well, when gluten and casein aren't adequately digested, they turn into substances with similar chemical structures as these opioid drugs. Unfortunately, some people with poor gut function are not digesting these opioid peptides efficiently, which is when they become toxic. They pass through the intestines into the bloodstream and then cross the blood–brain barrier and block certain areas of the brain, just like morphine and heroin would do (Campbell-McBride 2004).

There has been much scientific research linking high levels of gluteomorphins and casomorphin in the body to autoimmune disease, depression, anxiety, panic disorder, psychosis, autism and schizophrenia (Walsh 2012). Scientific studies into schizophrenic and autistic patients have shown an improvement in symptoms when dairy and gluten are removed from their diet.

I should point out that people with robust digestion are unlikely to suffer any ill effects from consuming gluten or casein. And even people with gut dysbiosis may tolerate gluten and casein just fine. And the percentage of people who suffer mental health issues after eating gluten and casein will be relatively low. Perhaps this is why it's not widely discussed (Woodford 2021).

Don't worry if you suspect you may be suffering the ill effects of gluten and casein consumption because I recommend cutting out both as part of the three-point plan. This may heal your gut to the point where you can reintroduce small amounts without any negative reaction. Remember to record and monitor your progress in your journal.

Interesting titbit

There has been some speculation that people with pale skin, red hair and freckles are more affected by gluten and casein sensitivity (Carolbetty 2009).

Sugar is not your friend!

Sugar is *everywhere*! It's in chocolate, cakes and sweets – and it's also a hidden ingredient in most processed foods such as breakfast cereal, white bread and ready meals. Sugar has often been described as 'pure, white and deadly', and this has never been truer than when applied to people with gut and brain symptoms. It's an inflammatory ingredient, and inflammation contributes to gut and brain symptoms (Jamar et al 2020).

Sugar isn't easy to digest and the body must use its vitamin and mineral reserves in order to metabolise it. Because the Western diet contains excessive amounts of sugar, vitamin and mineral deficiency is rife. Most of my clients are already nutrient deficient because of digestion and absorption issues, so I always strongly recommend they avoid foods that deplete their nutrient reserves even further.

Lactose is the predominant sugar in milk, and a large percentage of people are intolerant to it. So it follows that people may suffer from other forms of sugar maldigestion too. Fructose, the sugar found in fruit, tends to be tolerated by most of my clients because it's a mono sugar and therefore only requires minimal digestion. The conclusion I've come to is that refined sugar is extremely bad for you and is best avoided as much as possible.

Sweeteners

These are additives used as a substitute for regular cane sugar and can be found in so-called 'sugar-free' foods, which are big business. Originally aimed at diabetics, there's now a huge range of these foods on the market. Unfortunately, sweeteners are not easily digested or absorbed, and may cause diarrhoea, gas, cramps and bloating.

Sucralose is a popular sweetener that some studies have suggested is carcinogenic (cancer forming), neurotoxic and damaging to the gut microbiome (Schiffman 2023). So, for those who think they are doing themselves a favour by switching to sugar-free foods... think again!

Processed foods

Processing changes a food's chemical and biological structure. Fats are hydrogenated and a long list of chemicals are added, such as flavour enhancers, e-numbers, colours, preservatives, additives and solvents (Sambu et al 2022). The end result is a concoction of chemicals that shouldn't really be classed as a food. They're just designed to look and taste good. They're not designed for health and wellbeing. In fact, quite the opposite! Processed foods have many unhealthy fats and sugar added to them so they're extremely bad for your heart and your waistline. And they're just as bad for your gut microbiome. This is because processed foods feed the bad gut bacteria and encourage gut dysbiosis (Hrncirova et al 2019; Lane et al 2022). Processed foods are highly addictive. I'll make no bones about it – the food companies want you to become addicted! It's how they make their profit.

Processed foods are everywhere. They're considered the norm and are the staples of most people's diets. A few processed foods such as olive oil, canned fish, frozen fruits and vegetables, dried fruit, and hummus are OK to eat, though. When considering how healthy a processed food is, look at the ingredient list and ask yourself, could I make this at home? If the answer is no, don't buy it! The shorter the list of ingredients, the better. For example, some peanut butters are literally just peanuts and oil, whereas other brands have a long list of added chemicals and sugars.

Our bodies have not yet evolved to deal with processed foods. Instead, they're designed to digest whole foods in their natural state. So, can you see why some of the things you've been eating have upset your digestion? Please read *Ultra-Processed People* by Chris van Tulleken (2023). It's terrifying – but it will give you the willpower to avoid processed foods.

FODMAP foods

FODMAP stands for:

» Fermentable
» Oligosaccharides
» Disaccharides
» Monosaccharides and
» Polyols.

But these words are way too long and sound harder to understand than they actually are! They're more commonly known as carbohydrates. These particular carbohydrates can be difficult for the body to digest and absorb. As a result, they often sit in the gut and ferment, causing bloating, gas, constipation and diarrhoea (Nanayakkara et al 2016). These fermentable carbohydrates are not usually the cause of gut dysbiosis. In most cases, people develop dysbiosis for other reasons such as stress, antibiotic use or a poor diet, which then impairs the digestion of high-FODMAP foods. This is good news because it means that, if you remove the factors that triggered your gut dysbiosis and follow the three-point plan to heal your gut and improve your digestion, you should be able to tolerate high-FODMAP foods once again.

There has been a lot of scientific research done into the FODMAP diet in recent years (including the study cited above), and thousands of people are gaining tremendous relief from their digestive symptoms by following a low-FODMAP diet. In my experience, clients whose main symptoms are bloating, burping and severe flatulence feel much better when introducing the low-FODMAP diet. In fact, my windy clients tend to fare better when they decrease their consumption of *all* carbohydrates, not just FODMAPs.

A great success story

One of my clients was really struggling with chronic flatulence. Things were so bad he avoided going into the office to work and instead worked from home as much as possible. On the days he did go into work, he had to stop himself from trumping all day long, which made him severely bloated with terrible tummy aches. He didn't dare sneak out any trumps quietly in the office because they smelt so vile he was worried about gassing his colleagues! He said he remembered feeling so crippled by the trapped wind one day that he went to the gents' toilets at work and sat in a cubicle and cried. Poor chap! There's nothing worse than holding in your trumps – but nothing more satisfying than letting them out!

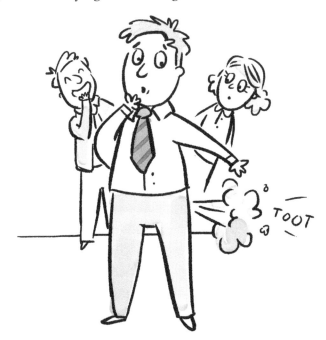

I met this client years ago, long before FODMAPs had been as thoroughly researched as they are now, so I didn't immediately recommend he cut them out. I just advised him to cut out dairy and gluten. Most of my clients see a reduction in their digestive symptoms within days, but after a fortnight, he'd only seen minimal improvement in his symptoms.

When I dug a little deeper into the exact ingredients he used in his home-cooked meals, I discovered he used tons of garlic and quite a lot of onion, which are both high in FODMAPs. I advised him to cut these out completely, and he felt so much better. The flatulence massively reduced, and it was much less stinky! But I was interested to know why he'd suddenly become so sensitive to these foods. He said the onset of symptoms coincided with his father's death. He described his grief as a pain that gnawed away inside him. I believe the stress and grief had upset the balance of his gut microbiome to the point where his poor tummy could no longer cope with digesting high FODMAP foods. I recommended he ask his GP to refer him for counselling to help him deal with his grief. He followed my three-point plan for several months to correct his gut dysbiosis, and the last time I spoke to him, he was feeling well and had reintroduced small amounts of garlic and onion back into his cooking with no ill effect.

Implementing a low-FODMAP diet

Let's take a closer look at high-FODMAP foods to understand which ones you may need to temporarily exclude from your diet. The list is quite long but here are some of the more commonly eaten: watermelon, nectarines, artichokes, garlic, onions, leeks, asparagus, lentils, Brussels sprouts, wheat, lactose, glucose, fructose, mango, kiwi, pears, apples, dried fruits and fruit juice concentrate.

Don't be disheartened. There are still lots of yummy foods out there that you're allowed to eat. Look back at the beginning of your journal when you first started recording your diet and see if the days when you felt bloated and windy were the days you'd eaten high-FODMAP foods. Now you know why you have been trumping so much!

Do you remember I said that FODMAP foods are all carbohydrates? In my experience, FODMAPs aren't the only type of carbohydrate to trigger digestive symptoms. I think carbohydrates in general, if ingested in large quantities, have the potential to cause gut symptoms such as bloating, wind and tummy aches. My clients all tend to fare better when they reduce their carbohydrate intake. Our modern-day diet is more carb-heavy than previous generations'. How many grams of carbohydrates do you reckon you eat a day? I try to stay below 50 grams. As a guide, there are roughly 12 grams of carbs in one slice of brown bread, 35 grams in one slice of pizza and 50 grams in one slice of chocolate cake. You can see how the carbohydrates soon add up!

Genetically modified foods

These foods have had changes introduced to their DNA in order to develop desired traits such as resistance to disease or a tolerance to pesticides. This is not a natural process and would never occur in nature, and this makes them unstable and potentially toxic (Dona & Arvanitoyannis 2009). Considering how slow the human digestive system is to evolve, we must ask, how capable is it of digesting and processing these novel organisms and what effect is it having on our delicate gut microbiome and overall physical and mental health? There are widely conflicting views on GM foods, with some countries restricting or completely banning their usage. But one thing is for sure: no one really understands the long-term effects of GM foods, and so to eat them is to be a human guinea pig. Let me share a few health concerns regarding GM foods.

GM foods are more likely to cause allergic reactions because some of the proteins they contain are completely novel and have never before been consumed by humans. GM foods also contain antibiotic resistance markers. This may make disease-causing bacteria resistant to antibiotics. Antibiotic resistance is already becoming quite a problem and GM foods are only adding to it. The British Medical Association has said: 'There *should* be a ban on the use of antibiotic resistance markers in GM foods, as the risk to human health from antibiotic resistance developing in microorganisms is one of the major public health threats that will be faced in the 21st century.'

(BBC News 2002) But as far as I'm aware, there still hasn't been a ban.

It's important to eat organic whenever possible because genetically modified organisms (GMOs) are prohibited in organic produce. Everyone should constantly choose nutrient-dense foods that are as close to their natural state as possible and avoid foods that can damage the gut microbiome. As a result, GM foods are not to be recommended.

The following list could contain GMOs unless labelled otherwise: corn and all foodstuffs containing corn, dairy products, potatoes, granola bars, soybeans, veggie burgers, margarine, protein powders containing whey, wholewheat bread, low-sugar foods and drinks containing aspartame.

Interesting titbit
Did you know that a genetically engineered bovine growth hormone is used to make cows produce more milk? It's called insulin-like growth factor 1 (IGF-1), which finds its way into the cow's milk and is then consumed by humans. It has been linked to breast, prostate and colon cancer (Perez-Cornago 2020).

Soya
A high percentage of the world's soya production is genetically modified and, as we've discussed, GM foods aren't particularly good for you. Soya is added to lots of processed foods. You can find it in infant milk formulas, baby foods, dairy replacements, vegetarian foods, margarine, dressings, sauces, biscuits, bread and pizzas.

A few years ago, soya suddenly became extremely popular when it was suggested that it lessened the severity of unpleasant menopausal symptoms in women from Eastern cultures (Chandler 2021). However, the type of soya eaten in the West varies greatly from the soya eaten in the East, where it's consumed in its natural state as a whole bean or fermented as natto, miso or tempeh. In this form, it has many health benefits. Fermented foods are especially good at redressing the balance of the gut microbiome.

The type of soya we eat in the West is called soy protein isolate. It goes through food processing, whereby the soybean fibre is removed using an alkaline solution. The beans are then soaked in an aluminium acid wash. Aluminium has been linked to Alzheimer's and dementia. After the wash, the soybeans are treated with other carcinogenic chemicals, so the end result isn't so much food but more of a chemical medley (Sukalingam et al 2015)! And, as we know, chemicals upset the microbiome and cause inflammation. I think I've banged on about inflammation and the importance of a healthy gut microbiome enough by now for you to understand just how crucial I think it is to your health and wellbeing. I hope I'm persuading you to avoid foods that damage your precious flora and fauna.

By this point in the book, I appreciate that you may be thinking, what on earth *can* I eat? But I promise you that not all the food groups I've mentioned will trigger your symptoms, though some of them probably will. It's just a process of discovering which ones. Bear with me!

Resistant starches

Many of the carbohydrates in your diet are starch. However, some starches function similarly to fibre and are resistant to digestion. Resistant starches are classed as a prebiotic because they feed your friendly bacteria, which positively influences the gut microbiome. However, resistant starches can irritate the guts of some people with gut dysbiosis. It's like some other foods I've mentioned: what may benefit one person irritates another. Gut and brain symptoms are such a personal thing. The following foods are high in resistant starch, so be aware when eating them and make a note of your reaction in your food journal: raw oats, cashews, green bananas, cereal products, rice, legumes, and foods that have been cooked and cooled or foods that have been reheated, particularly cooked and cooled potatoes.

Meat

I recommend my clients consume animal protein because it has many health benefits:

» Meat aids brain function because neurotransmitters, such as serotonin, tend to be made from amino acids, the building blocks of protein.
» Amino acids also help to regenerate and repair cells and tissues such as the gut wall.
» Meat aids bone strength.
» Meat contains vitamins and minerals.

But the quality and quantity of meat you consume is vitally important. Traditionally farmed animals are often fed grain, which you're trying to avoid. In addition, animals housed in poor conditions are automatically given antibiotics in their feed to keep infections at bay. This means that every time you eat meat, you too are consuming antibiotics (Ghimpeteanu et al 2022).

Animals are also given hormones and steroids, which you will then ingest. This is why, wherever possible, I recommend eating organic or pasture-raised meat. Pasture-raised animals are free to roam and their feed hasn't been treated with pesticides or chemical fertilisers. These animals naturally absorb more vitamins and minerals, which in turn benefits you. Look for a farm that guarantees their meat is both organic *and* pasture raised. I use Green Pastures Farm. You can order their food online, and it's delivered straight to your door. Pigs and chickens can't be grass fed but should still be raised outdoors and be free to forage. Pork contains higher levels of parasites than other meat, making it extra important to buy good quality organic meat.

Eating too much red meat causes inflammation and has been linked to constipation and bowel cancer. A fascinating book that looks at this is *The China Study* (2005), by T Colin Campbell, the author of more than 300 research papers and three books. *The China Study* is the most comprehensive study ever undertaken of the relationship between diet and the risk of developing disease and shows the dangers of a diet high in animal protein.

I usually have one or two meat-free days each week, just to give my digestion a rest. And on the days when I eat meat, I only eat small portions. A quick and easy way of working out how much meat you should be eating is that 70 per cent of your plate should be covered in vegetables and salad. Vegetables are alkalising, which means they help reduce inflammation. Too much protein is acid forming. The body neutralises this with sodium and calcium taken from bones. So, a high-protein diet may lead to calcium deficiency.

I recommend that you only eat wild-caught fish because it contains fewer chemicals and heavy metals than farmed fish. Unfortunately, our oceans are polluted, and so even wild-caught fish has risks. The trick is to make smart choices. Shellfish, mackerel and tuna tend to be more highly contaminated. Wild-caught salmon, cod, sardines, trout, sole and halibut are better choices. Find a good local fishmonger or, if you buy fish from the supermarket, it should say on the packet whether it's wild caught or farmed. If you eat a lot of fish, please take a selenium supplement because selenium is a mercury antagonist and will prevent mercury building up to toxic levels in your body.

Interesting titbit

Did you know that some cattle are fed chicken faeces? Someone had the bright idea that because chicken faeces contain protein, it would make a suitable food for cows. So, the cattle absorb the faeces and we end up eating the beef and dairy that contains traces of chicken faeces. It really makes you question what on earth we're eating! (Cullinan & Newey 2024)

Summing up

After reading the last few chapters, I hope you can understand the negative effects of these food groups and why I advise clients to exclude them. You'll know within a few weeks if excluding these foods is benefiting you. I recommend that you do this with the guidance of a nutritionist to ensure you're still eating a balanced and nutritious diet. I wanted to give you a thorough explanation of each food group so that you understand why I'm asking you to give them up. Hopefully, now that you understand their detrimental effects, it will give you the motivation and willpower to alter your diet. Panic not! There are plenty of healthy, nutritious foods still available for you to eat.

Eating a balanced diet

The table on page 138 will help you identify the best sources for each of the vitamins and minerals. Use it to help you find foods that you like, and which will give you variety.

Anti-nutrients

It's important to understand the effects of the foods you eat. Many of the common Western foods we eat are anti-nutrients. These are foods that contain few or no nutrients, and so they must draw on the body's store of vitamins and minerals to be metabolised and digested. If we eat these foods regularly, they deplete our vitamin and mineral status. Some of the common anti-nutrient foods include sugar, processed foods, dairy, gluten and alcohol (Levy 2018).

Food combining

This is based on the idea that certain foods digest well together while others do not. This is because different food groups are digested differently. For example, carbohydrate digestion begins in the mouth and continues in the small intestine. Protein, however, doesn't start being digested in the mouth. Instead, it requires the acid environment of the stomach and usually spends several hours there before being moved on. Our ancestors evolved by eating a mainly vegetarian diet with an occasional 'kill', which would have had to be eaten quickly before it went off. This means our digestive system hasn't evolved to digest protein and carbohydrates at every meal. Fruit is another food to be wary of combining. Fruit passes through the stomach quickly. If you eat it within an hour of consuming heavy protein that sits in your stomach for several hours, the fruit will also loiter in the stomach, where it will ferment and cause gut symptoms. The evidence to back up food combining is sketchy, but I thought it was worth mentioning because a lot of my clients have seen great improvements in their gut symptoms when they follow the food combining principles. Give it a go and see what you think.

Vitamin A	Red/yellow/orange fruit and vegetables, dark green leafy vegetables, egg yolk, cod liver oil, lamb's liver, spinach, broccoli
Vitamin D	Skin exposed to sun, dairy products, egg, herring, mackerel, salmon, oysters, cod and halibut, mushrooms
Vitamin E	Nuts, seeds, cold-pressed vegetable and nut oils, pine nuts, avocados, eggs, salmon, sardines, tuna, leafy greens
Vitamin C	All fruit and vegetables, in particular tomatoes, spinach, cabbage, broccoli, Brussels sprouts, cauliflower and red and green peppers
Vitamin B1	Potato, nuts, pulses, squash, asparagus, lentils, pork, beef
Vitamin B2	Meat, fish, mushrooms, spinach, almonds, avocados, eggs
Vitamin B3	Lentils, nuts, pulses, tuna, salmon, chicken, turkey, lamb, red meats, liver
Vitamin B5	Mushrooms, fish, avocados, sunflower seeds, lentils, nuts, pulses, eggs, meat
Vitamin B6	Green leafy vegetables, nuts, bananas, avocados, seeds, egg yolk, meat, fish
Vitamin B12	Fermented soya products (tempeh, miso), soy sauce, edible seaweed, black-eyed beans, eggs, oysters, sardines, tuna, shrimp, turkey and chicken, liver, organ meats
Folic acid	Green leafy vegetables, wholegrains, nuts, citrus fruits, mushrooms, dates, peanuts, root vegetables, sprouted seeds, black-eyed beans, eggs, liver, kidneys
Biotin	Mushrooms, nuts, cauliflower, cabbage, watermelon, sweetcorn, peas, tomatoes, milk, egg yolk, herrings, oysters
Essential fatty acids (EFAs)	Walnuts, seaweed, flaxseeds, hemp seeds, sunflower seeds, evening primrose oil, nuts and seeds, oily fish
Calcium	Green leafy vegetables, broccoli, nuts, seeds (especially sesame/tahini), pulses, yoghurts, tinned fish, including bones (anchovies and sardines)
Magnesium	Nuts, seeds, green leafy vegetables, buckwheat, beans, raisins, peas, soya, crab
Iron	Nuts, seeds, lentils, beans, spinach, pulses, dates, prunes, yoghurt, shellfish, red meat, liver, black pudding
Zinc	Pumpkin seeds, nuts, pulses, some vegetables, egg yolk, oyster, haddock, shrimp, red meats
Manganese	Nuts, pulses, green leafy vegetables, tea, pineapple, dark chocolate
Selenium	Walnuts, Brazil nuts, mushrooms, cabbage, courgettes, cheese, eggs, cod, oysters, tuna, herring, chicken, beef liver, turkey
Chromium	Green peppers, apples, mushrooms, asparagus, egg yolk, Swiss cheese, oysters, chicken, lamb, beef, poultry, broccoli

Part 2

The three-point plan

My three-point plan is a three-pronged approach to treating gut and brain symptoms.

» **Point 1 – Dietary changes:** This is all about removing foods that upset the gut microbiome and cause inflammation and fermentation, and replacing them with nutrient-dense whole foods.

» **Point 2 – Lifestyle factors:** A few small lifestyle changes can be all it takes to induce relaxation and reduce stress, or at least help you to manage stress. Stress is a major cause of gut and brain symptoms and may cause long-term damage to your gut microbiome, so incorporating a few of my lifestyle recommendations is an important part of your healing journey.

» **Point 3 – Supplements:** Nutritional supplements such as vitamins, minerals and probiotics are also an important part of your healing journey. The Western diet is extremely low in nutritious foods, leaving many of us deficient. Gut dysbiosis compounds the problem because an inflamed gut and a damaged microbiome hinder the absorption of vitamins and minerals from your food, leaving you deficient and requiring support from nutritional supplements.

I believe all three are essential for a return to full health. This approach to healing is holistic; it treats the cause of disease and puts you in control of your own health. It's a way of life that offers a long-term solution. My three-point plan can require a lot of motivation and effort on your part, but at some point, the cycle of rubbish food and rubbish health must end, and the only way to do that is with some tough love!

Chapter 9

Point 1: Dietary changes

Creating the perfect diet for you

OK, let's look at how to create the perfect diet and nourish yourself so that you heal and remain healthy for the rest of your life. My diet is designed to reduce inflammation and fermentation, rebalance the gut microbiome, reduce toxicity, heal and seal the gut, and improve brain and gut health. I recommend that you embrace wholesome, natural foods as a long-term way of eating because it's a worthwhile investment in your health and your future.

I realise I've bombarded you with information about all the different food groups that I think are bad for you, so I wouldn't blame you if you were in a blind panic thinking, 'What on earth can I eat?!' My aim was to give you a thorough explanation of each food group, so you understand why I'm asking you to give it up. Hopefully, now that you understand their detrimental effects, it will give you the impetus to alter your diet. Rest assured, in this chapter I'm going to be telling you about foods you *can* eat!

I'm not going to ask you to eat anything wacky or unusual. Instead, I'd like to take you back to basics. Imagine how your grandparents might have eaten: no processed foods, minimal sugar, less bread, more healthy fats. I call this style of eating 'eating clean'.

There's nothing fancy or clever about it. It's all about cutting out the rubbish. As I love to say, 'Eat rubbish, feel rubbish!' It's that simple. Unfortunately, the foods that I would class as rubbish have become the norm: fizzy drinks, coffee, sugary foods, chocolate, cake, bread. Bread is the clincher! I can see the panic in my clients' faces when I ask them to stop eating bread – but I promise it's possible to cut it out. There are some delicious alternatives. Most of what we eat is out of habit. It doesn't take long to develop new eating habits and for your tastebuds to adapt and start craving the new, healthier foods that you introduce into your everyday diet. Cutting out bread, dairy, sugar and processed foods doesn't mean you'll be missing out on any vital nutrients, because these foods are anti-nutrients. By cutting out these foods, you'll naturally find that you're filling up on healthier, more nutritious foods. I've lost count of the number of clients who have said to me, 'My digestion problems can't be caused by the food I eat because I eat a healthy, balanced diet.' And they genuinely mean it. But unfortunately, foods that you consider to be healthy might not agree with you.

A point worth making here is, if after a few weeks of eating clean, you feel no better, it's possible this method isn't for you. The vast majority of my clients soon notice an improvement in their symptoms when they follow the three-point plan. I usually find people have an idea of which foods trigger their symptoms, so trust your intuition. The biggest challenge is finding the willpower to stick to your new way of eating. Hopefully, now that you understand why all these foods are bad for you, it will give you the motivation you need. Prepare yourself for a struggle in the first few weeks. Some people make the transition easily, but others find it extremely difficult and regularly fall off the wagon. The thing to remember is that the more times you 'cheat' by indulging in your old favourite foods, the longer it will take for you to lose the taste and the craving for them. So, you're only prolonging the agony! I can promise you that your tastes will change, and instead of craving your usual lunchtime sandwich, you'll long for a plate of roasted vegetables or a salad.

Useful tips to help you on your way

Probably the hardest dietary change is giving up sugar. To help you beat your craving, try licking a lemon every time you get the urge for something sweet. It sounds disgusting, but it's not that bad, and it really does work.

Remember, digestion starts in the mouth, so take your time and chew well. This will start to break down the food and take some of the workload off your stomach.

The average stomach is roughly only the size of your clenched fist, so eating a portion any bigger than that causes overload, and your digestion will struggle to cope.

Try to stop eating before you feel full. Your digestion will improve, and you'll feel less bloated and uncomfortable.

Another useful tip when identifying foods that don't agree with you is that the foods we crave the most are usually the ones we are intolerant to. I know, it seems unfair, doesn't it?

Probably the most important tip I can give you is to wash fruit, vegetables and salad before eating to remove pesticides and other chemicals from your food. I advise soaking them in water with Himalayan sea salt for 20 minutes, or soaking them in water and vinegar for 20 minutes. Use one part vinegar to four parts water. After soaking, rinse them in running water before eating.

Read on to discover which foods you'll be avoiding and which foods you'll be enjoying.

Foods to avoid

- » refined carbohydrates
- » sugar
- » sweeteners
- » syrup
- » confectionery, all sweets, cakes, pastries, chocolate, etc
- » sugary drinks
- » sports drinks
- » soda drinks

- » shop-bought fruit juice
- » alcohol
- » coffee
- » canned fruit and vegetables
- » corn
- » grains
- » pasta
- » flour (apart from millet, coconut or almond flour)
- » all dairy products: milk, cheese, yoghurt, butter, etc
- » margarine
- » cereal, including breakfast cereal
- » baking powders (except bicarbonate of soda)
- » salted or roasted nuts
- » smoked meats and fish
- » processed meats: bacon, sausages, salami, packaged meats
- » other processed foods
- » ready meals
- » gravy
- » cashew nuts and peanuts (these usually contain traces of mould, which upsets the gut microbiome – see Levy 2024)
- » chewing gum
- » soya products
- » gluten
- » all cooking oils (apart from cold-pressed olive oil, avocado oil and coconut oil).

All the above foods have health drawbacks, as I have discussed in earlier chapters. So, even if your digestive system can tolerate them, I recommend you cut them out completely until your gut is healed and thereafter only eat them in moderation.

Foods to enjoy

- » herbal teas
- » freshly squeezed vegetable juice
- » natural honey (my favourite is manuka honey)

- » vegetables (preferably organic)
- » low sugar fruits – strawberries, blueberries, blackberries, raspberries, cantaloupe melon, occasional apples
- » salad
- » coconut yoghurt, coconut milk, coconut oil
- » almond milk
- » lentils and beans (in moderation because they may cause inflammation)
- » buckwheat, quinoa, amaranth (in moderation)
- » fresh nuts, except cashews and peanuts
- » nut butter (except peanut butter)
- » eggs
- » meats (preferably organic or pasture raised)
- » fish (preferably wild caught)
- » canned fish
- » olives
- » olive oil (organic and cold pressed)
- » cider vinegar
- » seaweed
- » ghee
- » dark chocolate, 75 per cent cocoa (small amounts).

In a nutshell, I would like your diet to consist of pasture-raised meats, wild-caught fish, vegetables, salad, low-sugar fruits and healthy fats. In addition, I'd like you to eat the full range of recommended foods rather than eating the same foods repeatedly.

Three-day sample menu
Day 1

- » Upon rising   Cup of fresh ginger and lemon tea
- » Breakfast   Poached eggs on almond bread
- » Snack   Strawberries, coconut yoghurt, almonds
- » Lunch   Chicken salad
- » Snack   Crudites dipped in guacamole
- » Dinner   Salmon served with vegetables

Day 2

»	Upon rising	Freshly squeezed vegetable juice
»	Breakfast	Wild-caught smoked salmon and avocado
»	Snack	Dark chocolate
»	Lunch	Homemade vegetable soup and almond bread
»	Snack	Homemade celeriac chips
»	Dinner	Homemade moussaka and green vegetables

Day 3

»	Upon rising	One mug of bone broth
»	Breakfast	Linseed porridge topped with raspberries
»	Snack	Hard-boiled egg dipped in Himalayan salt
»	Lunch	Chicken salad
»	Snack	Apple with a handful of walnuts
»	Dinner	Homemade lamb and vegetable curry with cauliflower rice

For those of you who are clued up on the various diets out there, you may recognise this way of eating as very similar to the paleo diet – also known as the caveman diet, the Stone Age diet or the hunter-gatherer diet. There are many scientific studies citing the benefits of the paleo diet (eg Fraczek et al 2021). It improves IBS symptoms, lowers inflammation, lowers cholesterol, lowers BMI, reduces waist circumference and blood pressure, and even reverses metabolic syndrome and type 2 diabetes. What's not to love?

This is the diet that our ancestors ate, and it caused them to evolve into a superior species. Therefore it's the diet chosen by evolution. It doesn't include any of today's major food allergens such as gluten, grains, dairy, sugar, soya and processed foods. These are 'new' foods. Well, they are to your genes and your digestion anyway. The paleo diet doesn't allow foods that only became available with the onset of farming. The theory behind this is that human genes haven't fully adapted to the dietary changes of the 10,000 years since the agricultural revolution. As such, they cannot tolerate 'modern' foods (Spreadbury 2012).

Hopefully, after reading my explanations about these foods in previous chapters, you understand why they aren't always good for us. The paleo diet is naturally low in carbohydrates, which is great for healing a fermenting gut and for keeping blood sugar levels and emotions stable. Some people make the mistake of filling up on protein when they follow a low-carb eating plan. But too much protein converts into sugars, which isn't good for anyone. Every time you sit down to a meal, I'd like three quarters of your plate to be taken up with salad and vegetables if these are foods you digest well.

The gut transforms plant foods into butyrate, which nourishes the gut microbiome and helps to relieve brain symptoms, suppressing inflammation, maintaining blood sugar levels and repairing the gut wall and the blood–brain barrier, so I recommend eating salad and vegetables in abundance (Sun et al 2016).

What you must remember is that as a person suffering from gut and brain symptoms, you should be eating with the intention of minimising these symptoms. It's all about finding a way of eating that suits you, and we're all so different and unique. So, use my recommendations as guidelines, not rules. Keep on reading and researching and explore the various diets in the excellent books I've recommended in the Resources at the end of this book. The more knowledge you have, the better your health is likely to be.

Just for the record, I really dislike the word 'diet'. It sounds rigid and restrictive and immediately makes me want to eat something naughty! So, although I think that the foods I recommend are similar to the way our cave-dwelling ancestors would have eaten, I'm by no means endorsing one particular type of diet. Play around with my recommendations and find what works for you.

I should point out that I'm not recommending this way of eating as a temporary elimination diet; I'm recommending clean eating as a permanent way of life. There are endless studies linking poor diet to all the major diseases, so I urge you to adapt my recommendations in a way that suits you and you feel you can stick to long term. Healthful, nutrient-dense foods are nature's medicine.

A note to vegans and vegetarians

Over the years, I've noticed that my vegan clients eat a lot of grains, and my vegetarian clients eat large amounts of dairy, both of which may antagonise gut and brain symptoms. The problem we have here is that no longer eating them leaves you with an extremely restricted diet. I recommend that my clients try a short experiment and cut out grains and dairy for a few weeks. This should be long enough to know if eliminating them lessens gut and brain symptoms. If you feel better and decide to exclude them long term, I recommend working very closely with a professional who can monitor your diet and ensure you're still getting an adequate supply of nutrients.

The ketogenic diet

Our ancestors who ate a paleo diet will have been in a state of ketosis for much of the time. This is a perfectly healthy state where the body produces ketones and uses them for energy instead of glucose. Ketones are a type of acid that your liver produces. Ketones in the blood or urine generally indicate that your body is using its backup source of energy – fats. This is what happens when you have a very low-carbohydrate diet or when you have periods of fasting in the same way that hunter-gatherers would have done. I don't think it's necessary to follow a ketogenic diet to lessen your digestive symptoms. I think lowering your carbohydrate intake is sufficient to prevent a fermenting gut. However, there's growing evidence that ketones are helpful in the treatment of mental illness, and I have seen excellent results in myself and my clients (Stone 2024).

The ketogenic diet and brain symptoms

The ketogenic way of life has a profoundly beneficial effect on mental health (Bai 2024). So, for those of you who are struggling with brain symptoms, I think it could help you to understand its principles. However, if you're struggling to get your head around the food and diet recommendations I've made thus far, then don't read this section for now. My recipe section is low in refined foods, which will automatically keep your blood sugars stable, so you will be benefiting.

Ketosis

During the process of digesting food, your body converts what you eat into glucose, and this is what gives you energy. But ketosis changes this process slightly. It's a natural and healthy state that occurs when the body uses fat for fuel instead of glucose. This happens when you're eating a low-carbohydrate, moderate-protein and high-fat diet. This way of eating isn't a million miles from the paleo diet. Ketones are made from fat in your body and healthy fats from your diet. They provide a steady source of energy, unlike glucose, which can fluctuate. Eating too many carbohydrates causes these fluctuations. This makes your blood sugar levels unstable and causes brain symptoms in some susceptible people. Unstable blood sugar levels have a scientifically proven link to both depression and anxiety (Penckofer et al 2012).

Studies have shown that ketosis also reduces both depression and anxiety (Sethi & Ford 2022). This could be because of its positive effect on the neuropeptides, which reduce anxiety and the fight or flight response. It also increases GABA, the calming neurotransmitter. It also reduces oxidative stress, which is linked to mental illness. Another reason ketosis improves mental health is because it lowers inflammation. Another bonus to the ketogenic diet is that it boosts immunity, making you less susceptible to viruses and infection.

To enter a state of ketosis, you have two options. Fasting for around 18 hours is the average time it takes for the body to start running on ketones. Alternatively, eat between 20 and 50 grams of carbohydrates a day. This forces the body to manufacture ketones as an alternative source of energy. Ketones are made from the breakdown of fats. So, ketosis literally turns you into a fat-burning machine, which is good news if you have a few pounds to lose. It also suppresses appetite, which I find really liberating!

As part of the three-point plan, I've recommended you cut out grains, processed foods and sugar, so you'll naturally be eating fewer carbohydrates. If you want to be more specific and count the number of carbohydrates you're eating, there are lots of helpful apps (and, of course, your food, mood and poop journal), which make keeping track of your carbohydrate intake a doddle. There are also handy little ketone test strips you can pee on, which measure whether or not you're in ketosis. If you struggle with brain symptoms, it might also be worth monitoring your blood sugar levels using something like Accu-Chek Mobile, which allows you to do regular finger-prick blood glucose tests. But if counting carbohydrates, peeing on strips and pricking yourself with needles sounds like too much hard work right now, then instead focus on keeping your blood sugar levels stable by eating every three hours and always adding healthy fats to any carbohydrate. For example, if you eat an apple, eat a handful of nuts too. If you eat a salad, drizzle olive oil over it. The healthy fat found in nuts and olive oil forces down your insulin levels and keeps your blood sugar stable.

The keto diet should be a clean way of eating. It's possible to stay in a state of ketosis while making poor food choices, but I can't stress enough the importance of eating 'clean keto' as opposed to 'dirty keto'. A diet of bacon, artificial sugars and lots of dairy may keep you in ketosis, but it won't heal your gut. In fact, it could damage it further, so be mindful that your poorly functioning gut may be the source of all your troubles and make your food choices wisely. If you stick to my recommendations of pasture-raised meats, wild-caught fish, vegetables, salad, berries, healthy fats and bone broth, you won't go far wrong.

We are evolutionarily adapted to thrive in a state of ketosis (Freese et al 2017). Our ancestors will have spent much of their time in ketosis because they ate a low-carbohydrate diet for much of the year, and they will have had periods of fasting in between hunts. Fasting triggers ketosis.

Compare that with today's diet, which is high in refined sugar and processed foods. Do you think our ancestors would have evolved into the superior species if they'd eaten today's Western diet? 'We are heading for an idiocracy,' says Professor Michael

Crawford, who is director of the Institute of Brain Chemistry and Human Nutrition. He predicts by 2080 that more than a third of the world's population will have a mental health disability (Food for the Brain n.d.).

So, look after your brain health! Eat lots of healthy fats such as fish oils, olive oil, coconut oil, linseeds and nuts. Eat a moderate amount of protein and lots of fresh berries, vegetables and salad.

Our bodies require fat and protein for survival, but they can survive quite happily on minimal carbohydrates. I'm not suggesting you cut them out completely, but it proves the point that they're not essential to our survival. The foods and recipes I recommend are all allowed on a ketogenic diet, as long as you monitor your carbohydrate intake to ensure you're staying in ketosis.

Case study

A woman in her forties came to me for a nutrition consultation to discuss her long-term symptoms of irritable bowel syndrome, anxiety, panic attacks and depression. She'd noticed that during flare-ups of IBS, her mental health symptoms worsened and she suspected the two could be connected. She tried to discuss this connection with her GP, but they didn't agree and told her, 'A poorly tummy is bound to make you feel anxious and depressed', despite her trying to explain that intuitively she felt her mental health symptoms were caused by her poor gut function and not simply a reaction to them. She had tried antidepressants, tranquillisers and talking therapy with little relief and was feeling highly motivated to take charge of her own health.

As part of my three-point plan, I often recommend that my clients start with a 24- to 72-hour bone broth fast to allow the gut to rest and heal. On her third day of drinking nothing but bone broth and water and avoiding food completely, she rang to tell me how incredible she was feeling. She described experiencing calmness and clarity, rather than her mind 'feeling like a kite being tossed around in the wind'. I explained that this was probably due to her entering ketosis. I'd briefly mentioned the possibility of entering ketosis but she'd forgotten because there's so much information to absorb in an initial consultation. So I gave her another, more thorough explanation.

When I saw her for a follow-up a few weeks later, she was still in ketosis and still feeling profound relief from her brain symptoms but only moderate relief from her digestive symptoms. When I looked at her food, mood and poop journal, I saw she had made the mistake that many people make when they're determined to stay in ketosis – she was eating too much meat, not enough salad and veg and zero fruit. As a general rule of thumb, I recommend my clients eat 50–100 grams of protein a day, depending on their activity levels. A cooked chicken breast contains around 50 grams. She was eating several times this amount. I explained that long term, this way of eating may be detrimental to her health and that cycling in and out of ketosis would probably bring her the same mental health benefits and be healthier long term. This is called metabolic switching. This means switching between using ketones for energy to using glucose and then back to ketones and so on (Mattson et al 2018). So, on the days you switch to burning glucose, you include more complex carbohydrates in your diet and on the days you burn ketones, you fast or eat 20 to 50 grams of carbohydrates.

I gave her all the information she needed and arranged to see her again in a month, but she cancelled the appointment. I understood why; she was so relieved to be free of her debilitating brain symptoms that she was frightened to come out of ketosis, so she had ignored my advice to cycle. Now, this felt like a tricky situation for me to handle. Obviously I can't force my clients to follow my advice, but I felt I had a duty of care to make sure her diet and long-term health were better after seeing me, not worse! And so I bought her a copy of a book that explained ketosis and metabolic switching and left it along with a little note on her porch. She contacted me to thank me and a few weeks later she messaged to say she had incorporated switching and was eating more salad, vegetables and low-sugar fruits and was still feeling a massive improvement in brain symptoms and also a big improvement in her digestive symptoms. Success!

Insulin resistance

Have you heard of insulin resistance? It's when your cells no longer respond properly to the insulin your body produces in response to the carbohydrates you eat. Insulin is a hormone made in your body that helps manage blood sugar levels. When you eat, it's insulin's job to balance your blood sugar levels by moving the sugar from your blood into your cells. But if you eat too many sugary, carbohydrate foods the cells get 'full' and they won't let in any more glucose. As a result, glucose piles up in your bloodstream and insulin is constantly pumped out to deal with the backlog. This is when the glucose in your bloodstream starts getting converted into fat! This is because your cells are no longer responding to insulin. This is known as insulin resistance, which leads to diabetes and a host of gut and brain symptoms – and it's reaching epidemic proportions (Seidell 2000)!

I like my clients with brain symptoms to be aware that insulin resistance has a profound effect on the brain. It alters mitochondrial function and dopamine turnover and is associated with anxiety and depression (Kleinridders et al 2015).

In my experience of chatting to my clients, they're all eating way more carbohydrates than is good for them. Their biggest carbohydrate intake is at breakfast time. Breakfast cereals, toast, croissants and porridge are all high in carbohydrates. I'm not saying porridge is bad for you, but I wouldn't recommend you eat it every day. The oats plus the milk and the topping of honey or fruit can easily take you over 50 grams of carbohydrates. I recommend my clients ideally stay under 50 grams of carbohydrates for the *entire day*!

Snacking is another issue for my clients. Crisps, confectionery and bananas are the popular snacks. But your average chocolate bar contains 50 grams of carbohydrates, a bag of crisps contains around 20 grams, and a banana can contain up to 35 grams, so you can see why your blood glucose levels might be high. Like porridge, bananas are good for you in moderation. I just like my clients to keep an eye on their overall carbohydrate intake.

Most of my clients make smart choices for lunch and dinner, and this confuses them into thinking their overall diet is balanced and healthy. But I would estimate that three quarters of my clients were eating more than 200 grams of carbohydrates a day when I first met them. This is a lot more than previous generations will have eaten (Bradley 2019). And the evidence is all around you. In the past three decades the prevalence of obesity has trebled in some countries (Tiwari & Balasundaram 2023). In my opinion, this is mainly due to processed, convenience foods, which are high in carbohydrates. This can be a controversial topic because some people believe fat is the problem, not carbohydrates. However, studies show that our total fat intake has decreased but heart disease, diabetes and obesity have increased. So, clearly, fat is not the problem here (Johnston et al 2014). This pattern of eating a lot of carbs might not be typical for you but it's a conversation I've had many times with many clients, so I thought it worth repeating here.

Case study

I asked 21 of my clients to test their fasting blood glucose using a little home test kit. Two were unknowingly diabetic and nine were pre-diabetic! I've been convinced for years that we're all eating way too many carbohydrates but even I was shocked by the results of my little experiment. I'm keen for my clients to keep their blood sugar levels stable because fluctuations in blood sugar can cause brain symptoms. The happy by-product of lowering carbohydrate intake is that along with lowering insulin levels and balancing blood sugar, it also lowers blood pressure, cholesterol and triglycerides. I've seen it in my clients time and time again, and it makes perfect sense. We aren't evolutionarily adapted to eat the large amounts of carbohydrates that we eat today and it's playing havoc with our systems. The key to health, in my opinion, is to moderate your carbohydrate intake to ideally no more than 50 grams a day. A helpful home test you can do is HbA1c. It's available from foodforthebrain. org and it measures how healthy your blood sugar levels have been over the past few months.

Summing up

Now that you understand the various food groups and why some of them aren't great for your health, it's time to put your knowledge into practice. The recipe section will give you ideas for a tasty, nutritious diet while excluding the main offenders. Probably the best advice I can give you is listen to your body and trust your intuition about which foods you tolerate and which foods you don't.

If you would like to adopt my recommendations as a long-term way of eating, feel free to do so. But as with any major change, I recommend consulting your GP first. Your food journal is crucial at this time to allow you and your doctor to monitor your progress and to allow them to see that you're eating a healthy, nutrient-dense diet and you're feeling physically and emotionally better as a result.

Some people worry they won't be getting all the nutrients they need if they exclude any food groups. This may be the case if you make poor food choices, but you'll see in the recipe section that the foods I recommend are all nutrient dense. Plus, you'll be taking supplements that will boost your vitamin and mineral status. Another bonus is when you remove all the not-so-good foods, your gut will be able to heal and repair and therefore you'll be able to absorb more nutrients. So, you see, you'll probably be absorbing more nutrients than you have in a long time! There seems to be an assumption that when you're eating whatever you fancy your diet will be 'balanced', and that if you cut out any food groups, you're at risk of becoming deficient. I would argue this point, but if you're worried about getting enough vitamins and minerals while you're following my three-point plan, I recommend you have some blood tests to check your vitamin and mineral status. This will tell you exactly what you're deficient in. You can then follow the three-point plan for six months and retest. In my experience, my clients' vitamin and mineral status always improves. But don't take my word for it. If you have concerns, this is something you can easily monitor yourself.

After a few weeks of following my three-point plan, you should see a reduction in your digestive and brain symptoms. If you don't feel any better, find a professional to work with you. Don't just keep cutting out more and more foods, because you could do more harm than good.

You may feel rough for the first few days of following my diet recommendations – headache, fatigue and nausea are all common. It's just your body detoxing. Drink plenty of water and, if necessary, electrolyte drinks. This soon passes, and most of my clients feel great when they adopt a healthier way of eating. Their digestive and brain symptoms diminish, they have more energy, their skin looks brighter, they sleep better, aches and pains vanish, and overall health improves. The improvement in your health will hopefully give you the motivation to stick to my three-point plan.

I truly believe that a clean diet of organic, low-sugar fruits, vegetables, salad, pasture-raised meats, wild-caught fish and healthy fats should be the gold-standard, long-term diet for everyone who wants to live a long and healthy life.

Chapter 10
Point 2: Lifestyle changes

This is not as scary as it sounds, and doesn't involve doing anything too dramatic! The suggestions I'm about to make are more life-enhancing and aim to encourage you to make a little time for yourself to improve your physical, emotional and spiritual health. So, read through the following section and pick out the parts that most appeal to you.

It's easy to get caught up in the hectic pace of life, rushing from one task to the next, looking after everyone else's needs and neglecting our own. We no longer hear our body crying out to us for love and attention until we reach a crisis point such as an emotional or physical illness, and we're left looking in the mirror at a stranger, thinking, 'Who am I?' How did I get so out of touch with *me*? But you can stop this downward spiral by remembering to take time out for yourself and realising you're more than a wife, a husband, a parent or an employee. You are your own person. And it's important to have time alone in order not to lose sight of that fact, and just as important not to feel guilty for taking time for yourself. I once heard someone say, 'Love and care for yourself as if you are your only child.' I think this is extremely sound advice, and I regularly remind myself of it. Simple things such as taking a bath in candlelight, going for a walk in a park or spending time on a hobby or activity that gives you pleasure are all valuable and life-enhancing because they give your body and mind a chance to relax.

This is an extensive section and making lifestyle changes is a very personal thing, so not everything I suggest will resonate with you. Just look for something that you think will lower your stress levels and you can regularly incorporate into your daily routine.

Human diet and lifestyle evolution

Our ancestors were hunter-gatherers. They foraged for plants and hunted animals. Their lives revolved around food. Hours a day will have been spent hunting and foraging. They were connected to nature and were dependent on each other, working together in a tribal community. Compare our ancestors' simple diet and lifestyle with the way we live today (Alt et al 2022). There really is no comparison! 'Civilisation' has led us further away from nature and our natural selves. Is there any wonder our digestion and mental health are in turmoil? We have sanitation, healthcare, education, supermarkets and food choices. We live in an era that mankind has looked forward to and worked towards for generations. In many ways, we live in paradise. So, why are there so many mental and physical health problems and so much unhappiness? We should be super-duper healthy and jumping for joy, shouldn't we? But unfortunately, we're not!

The Western way of life today is physically and emotionally unhealthy in many ways. The average 'normal' life looks something like this: in debt, living hand to mouth, feeling stressed and isolated; not doing enough exercise; a medicine cabinet full of painkillers, anti-depressants and indigestion tablets; a pressured, unrewarding job that funds a life that we're not really enjoying. This kind of lifestyle is like a nightmarish merry-go-round. And so, what do we do? We attempt to fill the emptiness we feel inside with dopamine hits from alcohol, binge eating, shopping, or more 'likes' on social media.

Sadly, this existence is the norm for many people. But you're not meant to just exist and barely get by. You're meant to thrive!

Prolonged unhappiness and disconnection are stressful, and as we all know, stress leads to poor mental and physical health. But don't blame yourself if you're feeling below par. As a wise person once said, 'It is no measure of health to be well adjusted to a sick society.' And unfortunately, the society we serve is sick. War, tyranny, poverty, food banks, corruption, dogma and struggle have become accepted norms. On a spiritual level, the life I've just described is empty and lacking. And on a physical level, it's downright unhealthy.

So, how can we solve this mini existential crisis? I think the solution has several layers. First, you must desire change. Many people don't want to step off the nightmarish merry-go-round because they find comfort in its predictability. But to free ourselves, we need to consciously choose a clean-eating, clean-living way of life. And on a spiritual level, we need to find a purpose in life and be connected to other people.

There are various ways to experience this connection, such as following a religion or spiritual practices. Having faith in something bigger than ourselves helps to give us a sense of purpose and peace. As an interesting aside, many of the world's most successful people – athletes, businessmen and women – have a strong faith that seems to help them tap into a higher power within themselves. However, I realise that religion is a turn-off for many people, so if spirituality isn't for you, then a practical way of experiencing connection and purpose might be through volunteer work. Find a cause you're passionate about. Working alongside like-minded people and contributing to society can be hugely beneficial for your wellbeing. Or, take up a team sport. If you're more of a loner, then walking in nature could be a way for you to experience a connection to yourself and the Earth.

Make time to do the things you love and spend time with people who uplift you. Having a loving community around you is so important for robust mental health. Conversely, loneliness and isolation are proven to be predictors of early death. The simpler your life and the more you can experience love, purpose and connection with yourself and others, the more joyful your life will be and the healthier in mind, body and spirit you will become.

What's the purpose of life? What's the purpose of *your* life? My purpose is to heal and free myself and to help other people to heal and be well and free. When you heal yourself, you become a healer. I would love this to become your purpose too, and together we can start a wave of healing that lifts the collective consciousness. That's my dream and the purpose behind writing this book. How wonderful if together we could change the paradigm away from a pharmaceutical approach to mental illness and instead be masters of our own health and happiness by approaching things from the angle of cause and prevention. Wouldn't that be empowering?

It's impossible to go back to the way our ancestors lived centuries ago, and let's be honest, we wouldn't really want to! But I would strongly recommend getting back to basics wherever possible. Live in line with the laws of Mother Nature. Slow your pace of life, live consciously and on purpose. Nourish and care for yourself and others. Cook whole foods from scratch and be mindful as you eat. Chew thoroughly and really taste your food and feel gratitude. There's a world of difference between lovingly preparing and eating whole organic foods to mindlessly scoffing fast foods in front of the TV. If you approach your health and my three-point plan from a place of love and with a sense of purpose rather than an attitude of deprivation, it will give meaning to your journey.

I believe we're all connected, so when you nourish and care for yourself, you benefit everyone. I appreciate you haven't bought this book for a lecture on how to live your life, but all I can do is tell you about the things that have benefited my life and my clients' lives. I hope the following section on lifestyle changes guides you to your own equilibrium.

One of the best books I've been recommended to read is *Twelve Steps and Twelve Traditions* by Bill Wilson (1952), which is given to recovering addicts at Alcoholics Anonymous. It guides you in how to live the life I've just described. The first time I read it, I was blown away at the love pouring out of every page. It wasn't at all what I imagined. It's like a beautiful guide to living a beautiful life and I think it should be compulsory reading for everyone, regardless of addiction. I regularly recommend the companion book, *The Twelve Steps and Twelve Traditions of Overeaters Anonymous* (2018), to my clients who are struggling to follow my dietary recommendations.

Environmental factors

When assessing your health and lifestyle, it's important to consider environmental factors because they contribute to disease and may well worsen your symptoms. Factors include diet, the area where you live, stress, pollution, illnesses and infections, medications, household cleaning products, cosmetics and much more.

This may sound a bit pessimistic, and you could be thinking, 'How on earth do I avoid all these environmental factors? They're everywhere!' But I think it's helpful and empowering to be aware of all the things that can compromise your health because then you can choose to avoid them wherever possible. Pollution, chemical exposure and processed foods are all on the increase, so it's no coincidence that inflammatory bowel disease, mental illness, food allergies, cancer, heart disease, autism and Alzheimer's are all increasing at a similar rate. Modern-day diseases should be renamed human-made diseases. Be aware of the detrimental environmental factors in your life and reduce them if you can. For example, ideally don't exercise near busy roads, eat organic foods and switch to non-toxic cleaning brands and cosmetics. A good rule of thumb when choosing your personal care products is: if you can't eat it, then don't put it on your skin!

Interesting titbit

According to a study published in 2008 (Anand et al), 5–10 per cent of cancer cases are genetic but 90–95 per cent are caused by environmental and lifestyle factors such as air pollution, cigarette smoking, fried foods, red meat, alcohol, obesity and physical inactivity. Just read that again: 90–95 per cent of cancers are caused by factors that are preventable!

The mind–body connection

It's well known that the mind–body connection exists. For example, if we feel embarrassed, we blush; or if we feel frightened, our heart beats faster. My clients with gut and brain symptoms often find that worrying about their illness makes their symptoms worse. Of course, the mind–body connection can work to your advantage as well as your disadvantage. It's possible to learn to control anxious thoughts and replace them with peaceful, calm ones. For this, I strongly recommend meditation. It has helped me and my clients tremendously in regaining control of both mind and body. It has helped me to hold on to my inner peace and serenity, even in the most trying situations. The key to meditation is practice and perseverance. It takes time to develop the habit of peace rather than the habit of worry.

You could compare the stressed, overanxious mind to an out-of-shape body. The body gets flabby and out of shape through eating unhealthy foods and not exercising, and the mind gets flabby and out of shape when we constantly indulge ourselves in negative thoughts and worries. It's important to remember who's in charge of your mind. You are! And you *can* choose what you think about. You can exercise your body and get it back in shape, and it's just the same with the mind. Its condition can be improved by regularly thinking positive, peaceful thoughts on purpose.

In my job as a nutritionist and reflexologist, I often take on the role of an unofficial counsellor. I once had a client who consulted me about a long list of ailments. She was a poorly, unhappy woman and seemed unable to comply with my three-point plan. One day, she tearfully opened up to me about a fallout with her sister that she felt terribly guilty about. We chatted and she decided that the only way she could ever find peace of mind was to apologise to her estranged sister. She later told me her sister had been delighted to hear from her and they healed their rift. My client's physical and emotional health immediately and miraculously started to improve without any other therapeutic interventions. Coincidence? Quite possibly.

Or perhaps it's further proof of the mind–body connection. I'll let you make up your own mind.

I believe that because the mind and body are intimately connected, we can't truly heal one without the other. An interesting follow-up to this case study is that it wasn't until *after* she reunited with her sister and her health improved that she implemented my three-point plan. She began taking much better care of herself in all aspects of her life. Her diet improved, she took her supplements religiously, she joined a weekly Zumba dance class, and went back to church after years of absence.

Positive thinking

The power of positive thinking can't be underestimated. How can you ever feel really well while thinking negative thoughts? What do you think causes you to feel stressed and unhappy? Is it the situation you're in, your thoughts about the situation or the way you think about yourself? Consciously and constantly weed out negative thoughts. By that, I mean every time a negative thought floats into your mind, acknowledge it and then purposefully replace it with a happy, positive thought. It's always handy to have some mood shifters up your sleeve. Mood shifters are things that will shift your thoughts from negative to positive. When you find yourself worrying, purposefully switch your attention to a happy memory, thoughts of a loved one or a daydream about places you'd like to visit.

My own personal mood shifter is to practise an attitude of gratitude. I must say 'thank you' 100 times a day. Thank you for running water into my home. Thank you for my healthy body. Thank you for my cosy bed. Thank you that I live in a free country. I even say thank you to my feet every day!

A common theme of negative thinking is to think critical thoughts about ourselves, but we should never get angry because of our imperfections. Having faults is a normal part of being human. Do you ever think, 'What's wrong with me?' Let me tell you, there's nothing wrong with you. And I know that without even meeting you! I think the society we live in, with social media and celebrity culture, sets unrealistic expectations. We feel that our own lives are pointless in comparison. If you can relate to these feelings, I recommend you read a book called *The Subtle Art of Not Giving A F*ck* by Mark Manson (2016), which became a *New York Times* bestseller. It advises us in a funny and uplifting way how to accept our flaws. If you need a gentle slap, this is the book for you!

Worry is one of the biggest thieves of joy, and we all know it's a complete waste of time. Worry is a vain attempt to try to control future events by thinking about them. So, do yourself a favour and be at peace with the things you can control and let go of the things you can't do anything about. It's worth considering why human behaviour often tends towards worry and anxiety. I believe it's an ancient animal instinct we have for survival. In our modern-day lives, we don't need to worry about predators or foraging for food. So, instead, we worry about financial pressures, employment, our children's welfare. This often manifests itself in depression, panic attacks, migraine and digestive problems. It's completely normal to experience stress. It's your inbuilt survival instinct kicking in. Just ensure you manage it and don't let it overwhelm you.

Subconscious behaviour

Some of our behaviours and beliefs are subconscious, and I'd just like to highlight a subconscious behaviour I've noticed in several of my clients. Some people thrive on their ill health and wear their ailments like a badge of honour. In a funny way they actually enjoy it. I know this will sound odd to many of you. After all, why would anyone choose to be poorly? However, being poorly fills a need for some people. Perhaps it's a need for attention or perhaps an excuse to avoid work and social situations. This need for illness will only apply to a small percentage of readers, but it's worth considering. Ask yourself, am I ready to feel well? And if the answer is no, ask yourself what need is illness fulfilling and could your needs be met in a healthier way?

Your personal paradigm

A large percentage of our thoughts and behaviour is habitual and is probably the result of our life experiences, and it affects the way we view ourselves and the world. But to be truly healthy, you need to consciously improve your day-to-day thoughts and habits. Your daily routine will have to change from the way you're currently living to something similar to my three-point plan. Be aware that your paradigm will constantly try to pull you back to your old, habitual ways of eating, thinking and living. But conscious action and repetition will form new neural pathways. So, the longer you follow my three-point plan, the more your self-image will change for the better. Just be prepared for your paradigm to put up a royal battle!

A great book to help you is *Change Your Paradigm, Change Your Life* by Bob Proctor (2021). Bob was a genius who helped millions of people make a success of their lives. His teachings will help you to become the person your goals and dreams require you to be.

Stress

Stress is a great example of the mind–body connection. Emotional stress can manifest in a host of physical symptoms: headaches, migraines, eczema and muscle pain can all be triggered by stress, as can gut and brain symptoms. What exactly happens to our digestion when we're stressed? In bygone times when the biggest stress for a cave dweller was running away from a grizzly bear, the body would go into fight-or-flight mode. This causes the digestion to temporarily shut down and stop working, so all the body's energy can be utilised to fight or flee (Harvard Health Publishing 2019). Unfortunately, our bodies can't distinguish between the stress of being chased by an angry bear or the stress of being stuck in a traffic jam, meaning we're constantly dipping into fight-or-flight mode unnecessarily.

Stress and gut dysbiosis are closely entwined and can become a vicious cycle. So, if you remove the stress, the unpleasant gut and brain symptoms should disappear, right? Unfortunately, this is easier said than done. Sometimes it will be possible to remove life pressures, but some stresses, such as work or an ill relative, are long term or permanent, so it's probably more practical to look at how you deal with stress. It's possible to manage your stress effectively; it just takes a little practice. Stress is complex, so we need a toolbox of different techniques to help us cope in different situations. I would strongly urge you to try some of the natural coping techniques I'll be recommending in this chapter before reaching for medication such as antidepressants, because they can have side effects that are more unpleasant than the original symptoms. That said, there are no prizes for being a brave soldier, so if you feel you really need it, then just see medication as a short-term helping hand while implementing natural stress management strategies.

Whenever a client tells me that stress makes their gut and brain symptoms worse, I always ask what stimulants they're consuming regularly. These people seem to be particularly sensitive to caffeine, sugar, alcohol and food additives. I always recommend my clients avoid eating while feeling particularly stressed. The body simply can't digest when it's in an emotionally stressed state, so I recommend a fresh vegetable juice instead of a meal and waiting until you've relaxed before eating again.

Case study

A client of mine had taken on a high-pressured job, which involved working away from home. He soon started experiencing panic attacks and digestive symptoms. I threw my whole toolbox of tricks at him: diet changes, supplements, meditation, massage, yoga. He also visited his GP, who prescribed tranquillisers – but all to no avail. I heard through his wife that he eventually suffered a nervous breakdown and was off work for over a year. I think this case study highlights the very real danger of stress and the profound effect it has on our mental and physical health. So, although this case study was not a success for me, I felt it important to share it with you. If you can relate to this story, I strongly urge you to walk away, if at all possible. No job is worth sacrificing your mental and physical health for.

Time management

In an era of modern conveniences, how are we so time poor when we should be time rich? I think the answer is that because everything is instant, we try to cram too much in. Emails and phone calls can be answered anywhere, so work intrudes into home life. Because we have so many opportunities, we may feel we have to be and do everything. This is great but only if we can get the balance right – and balance in life is so important. Gone are the days when life was slow and simple. Nowadays, we must make a conscious effort to keep things slow and simple. We seem to be more harassed and exhausted than ever before. Learn to delegate and let go of control wherever possible and above all, take your time!

I find planning my day with a to-do list helps me to use my time effectively – and I avoid multitasking. My female clients and friends all seem to be multitaskers – I think they feel as if they're getting things done quicker, but I'm convinced the opposite is true! Apart from anything else, it's stressful trying to do several things at once. So, focus on one thing at a time and give it your full attention.

Saying no

Many of us are people-pleasers, but this doesn't serve us. And, in quite a lot of cases, it doesn't serve the person you're trying to please, either! As soon as you feel you're being put upon, you need to back off a little. Give yourself boundaries and permission to say no to people without feeling guilty. It's impossible to please everyone. The truth is, not everyone is going to like you, and that's OK. I heard a statistic that around 10 per cent of the people we meet will not like us, so it's pointless running around trying to please everyone because not everyone will appreciate it. If saying no to people is something you struggle with, I would highly recommend polishing up on your assertiveness skills. The best way to do this would be to read a book or attend a short course.

Mindfulness

Mindfulness exercises are all about paying attention to the present moment, using things such as yoga, walking, meditation and breathing. They train your mind to keep your attention fully in the present moment. When you're stressed, it's common for your mind to become fixed on your worries or your thoughts to be running ahead, thinking of all the jobs that still need to be done that day. This scatters your energy and exhausts you. I use mindfulness to bring my energy into the present moment by focusing on all my senses in turn. For example, if I'm washing up the pots, I would become aware of the warmth of the water, the smell of the washing-up liquid, the sound of the birds singing outside, and so on. Whenever my mind starts running away with me, I bring my attention back into the room, become aware of my feet on the floor, and work my way through the awareness of my different senses again. I find it has an instant calming effect on me. Practised in this manner, mindfulness can easily be incorporated into your everyday life.

The Wim Hof Method

You may have heard of Wim Hof (aka The Iceman) from his TV series, *Freeze the Fear* (2022). His method of cold-water exposure and breathing exercises can offer a gateway to energy, peace and healing. He has thousands of testimonies from people who have freed themselves from the symptoms of multiple sclerosis, arthritis, mental health problems, addictions and many more conditions, all from following his breathing and cold-water method (Almahayni & Hammond 2024). It works by putting you back in control of your body and mind – and with control comes freedom. I feel a little concerned when describing Wim Hof that my words can't do justice to this man and his methods. His profound message of love and hope are probably best understood by reading his book, *The Wim Hof Method* (2020). Cold-water exposure isn't appropriate for everyone so do seek medical advice if you are in any doubt.

Eating in a relaxed manner

This is an essential part of good digestion. It has become the norm to eat in a hurried manner, quite often doing something else at the same time as eating, but this impairs digestion and absorption. So, for this reason, don't eat when you're feeling particularly stressed and uptight because you can just about guarantee you'll end up with indigestion.

If you can, sit down at every mealtime and give your full attention to enjoying your food. Eating meals is a great time to practise mindfulness. Try it and see how enjoyable mealtimes are when you really focus on the tastes, textures and smells. I like to start every mealtime with a little prayer of thanks to the food I'm about to eat and my digestive system for perfectly digesting my food.

Start each meal with three deep, slow breaths, and as you breathe out, focus on relaxing your stomach muscles. If the tummy muscles are tense while eating, this can cause spasms in the gut, usually resulting in tummy ache and possibly diarrhoea. Breathe in to the count of four, hold for four and then breathe out slowly to the count of eight. This will automatically activate your parasympathetic nervous system, switching you from fight-or-flight to rest and relaxation. This is a great little breathing exercise you can do anywhere, anytime to lower your stress levels.

If you wolf down your food without chewing properly, it makes it harder for the stomach to break it down, and this causes gas and bloating. So, chew, chew, chew! Did you know that chewing has been shown to reduce stress? This is why chewing gum is a proven relaxation technique (Smith 2016). Chewing your food thoroughly has the same relaxing effect. Try it and you'll see what I mean.

Sleep

A good night's sleep is incredibly important for your health. We think of sleep as a time when everything shuts off as we drift off to la-la land. But this is not the case. Sleep is a very active time when lots of important functions take place and our bodies need this time to repair and rejuvenate. In a perfect world, we would be sleeping around seven or more hours a night. But how many of us are getting that much sleep? In my experience the answer is not many! But don't get too hung up on the numbers because everyone is different and will need different amounts of sleep to function well.

If you feel you're not getting enough sleep, then take a 20 to 30-minute siesta or power nap during the day. Countless scientific studies (including a recent one by University College London) have shown the health benefits of a power nap (Gerretsen 2024). I usually combine my nap time with meditation. I generally meditate for ten minutes and then nap for ten minutes. If you can't nap because you're at work, a ten-minute meditation session is just as restorative.

You can do many things before bed to help aid a good night's sleep, such as disconnecting yourself from the internet and connecting with yourself with a good book or journal. I love meditating before going to sleep and find it helps me to drift off.

Be mindful of the stimulants you're eating and drinking before you go to bed and when the last meal of the day is. What you don't want is your digestive system to be busy at night because this will block other important functions such as detoxification and mitochondrial repair. For this reason, it's important not to eat anything for three hours before bedtime.

Try to go to bed and wake up at a similar time each day to regulate your circadian rhythm. Avoid artificial light during the night because it impairs melatonin and serotonin. And remember to put your mobile phone on airplane mode before you go to sleep (Baranwal et al 2023).

Meditation

In my experience, meditation is the most powerful and effective way to achieve deep relaxation. Meditation is preventative medicine at its best. It has been practised for thousands of years in different cultures and religions as a way of reaching new levels of consciousness. Fortunately, meditation is becoming trendy again, and classes are popping up everywhere. Science backs up what practitioners have known for centuries, which is that regular meditation calms the stress and anxiety part of the brain and helps new neural pathways of relaxation to form (Jamil et al 2023).

I was fortunate to have a forward-thinking GP, the lovely Dr Faire, who taught me to meditate when I was a teenager, and I'll be forever grateful because it's been a life-changing blessing. Meditation can be tricky to master because the mind tends to wander. The secret to success is not to get cross and frustrated with yourself. Instead, just gently keep bringing your mind back into the room and focus again on your breath. The groundwork is worth the time and effort because once you've mastered meditation, it's relatively easy to slip into that state of deep relaxation and expanded consciousness. A good way to get to grips with meditation is to start off by sitting for five minutes and focusing on your breathing. There are also some great apps you can download which are dedicated to meditation.

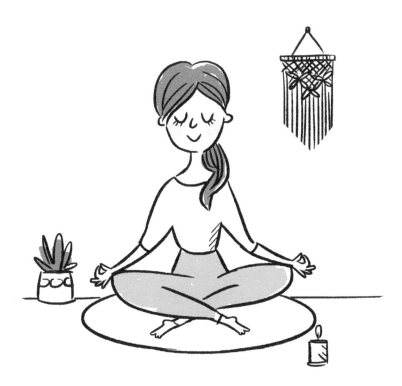

Relaxation exercise

Choose a time when you're unlikely to be disturbed. A warm environment with low lighting promotes physical relaxation. Perhaps you could choose some relaxing background music. Sit or lie in a comfortable, open position. Bring your attention into the room and become aware of each of your senses in turn. What can you hear? What can you feel?

Next, focus on your breathing. Correct breathing is essential for relaxation. Breathe in through your nose and out through your mouth. Try to make your out-breath a little longer than your in-breath. Next, silently say the word 'calm' to yourself as you exhale. Do this at least ten times and then pull your toes up towards your head. Hold for a couple of seconds and then release. Push your toes down towards the floor; hold and then release. Stretch out your legs, hold and then release. Tighten your tummy muscles, hold and then release. Clench your fists and stretch out your arms; hold and then release. Lift your shoulder blades towards your ears, hold and then release. Screw up your facial muscles and then release. Finally, imagine your spine relaxing and lengthening and your whole body becoming limp and heavy. Now, lie quietly for five minutes, focusing on your breathing or visualising a special place such as a beach scene or somewhere that holds happy memories for you.

A 12-minute meditation is available to listen to on my website, www.joannemordue.com

Breathing

Breathing plays an important role in digestion. But how many of us breathe correctly or even know the difference between good and bad breathing? Stress can speed up breathing, and we find ourselves almost gasping for air and taking in more oxygen than we require. This overload of oxygen perpetuates feelings of stress and causes digestive disturbances. Correct breathing is vital to our overall wellbeing. I would urge anyone to take the time to practise breathing exercises because the body can retrain itself so that deep, full breaths become a healthy subconscious habit.

To practise correct breathing, sit up straight or lie down on your back and take a moment to relax and ensure there's no tightness or tension in your body. Imagine that your torso is made up of three balloons sitting one on top of the other. In your tummy is a red balloon; on top of that and level with your diaphragm is a yellow balloon; and on top of that and level with your chest is a green balloon. Now breathe deeply into your red balloon, then your yellow balloon and finally the green balloon, filling them completely. Then breathe slowly out, ensuring the out-breath takes longer than the in-breath, emptying your chest first, then your diaphragm and finally your tummy. Then, push out the last remaining dregs of air before repeating the exercise again. With practice, this will become one continuous breath that will take roughly to the count of five to breathe in and to the count of eight to breathe out. The in-breath should be through the nose, and the out-breath can be through the nose or the mouth. I recommend practising this every day.

Gut dysbiosis and hyperventilating

Hyperventilating is rapid, shallow breathing. The excess oxygen can make you feel very peculiar with symptoms such as dizziness, cramps, stomach ache and panic. People with gut dysbiosis often experience hyperventilation because a bloated abdomen can put pressure on the lungs, making it difficult to take a deep breath. Several of my clients have told me they have woken in the night hyperventilating. This usually happened after eating a late dinner.

The best technique to calm your breathing is to gently cup your hands or a paper bag over your mouth and focus on lengthening your out-breath by letting out a long sigh. Try not to panic. I know it's frightening to lose control of your breathing, but it can't hurt you. The long-term solution is to reduce gut and brain symptoms by following the three-point plan and regularly practising abdominal breathing, as described above.

Exercise

The body needs to move! Exercise is extremely important for mental and physical health, so take the time to find an exercise that you enjoy and can regularly incorporate into your lifestyle. Exercise internally massages the gut, regulates bowel movements and improves physical and mental wellbeing. Try walking, swimming, resistance training, exercise classes or yoga.

Inactivity causes the gut to become sluggish. Bear in mind that regular exercise is part of human evolution. We're designed to be active, yet we're becoming more and more sedentary with each generation. There are many studies showing that exercise is an effective treatment for mental health and wellbeing (Mahindru et al 2023). If you haven't been physically active for some time, gentle, steady progress is key. Be careful not to overdo it at first.

Walking is often a good exercise to start with, or something simple such as putting on your favourite music and dancing around the house! Whatever form of activity you choose, pick something you enjoy and doesn't feel like a chore.

Complementary therapies

These are ancient healing techniques designed to restore health and equilibrium and include aromatherapy, reflexology, acupuncture and many more. The various complementary therapies have healed generations of people with a diverse range of ailments. Unfortunately, due to lack of funding, there has not been enough scientific research into proving the efficacy of complementary therapies. However, most of them are hundreds of years old and have been tested over time. As such, there's plenty of anecdotal evidence out there. Ask around and I'm sure you'll find people willing to share their success stories.

There's some suspicion in Western culture regarding complementary therapies. We like things to be scientifically proven. If they aren't, some people are quick to discredit them or label them as quackery. I remember about 20 years ago when scientific researchers declared they had proved acupuncture worked and it would now be available on the NHS. It was all over the news, and I remember shouting at the TV, 'Of course it damn well works – it's been healing people for hundreds of years!'

Complementary therapies are like Western medicine in that they sometimes work for you and sometimes they don't. It's just a case of finding the right therapy for you. But the great thing about alternative therapies is they rarely have side effects, and if they do, they're extremely mild. Complementary therapies aren't intended to replace conventional medicine, but they work beautifully alongside it. It's heartwarming to see aromatherapists working in hospices and acupuncturists working in doctors' surgeries.

I have my own personal homoeopathy success story. I used to suffer from eczema. Sometimes it was so severe, it would become infected. It was itchy, unsightly and sometimes downright painful. My doctor prescribed steroid cream, but it didn't help much – probably because it only suppressed the symptoms. When I was in my twenties, I visited a homoeopath and after only one treatment my eczema cleared up completely and has never returned. Over the years, I've recommended homoeopathy to many people struggling with eczema, and the majority have had great results.

Unfortunately, homoeopathy is still considered quackery by some people, but did you know that most of our modern-day pharmaceutical drugs are synthetic copies of plants (Gurib-Fakim 2006) and that many prescription drugs contain active ingredients derived from plants? For example, the main ingredient in digoxin, a heart medication, is extracted from the foxglove plant. The painkilling drugs morphine and codeine are derived from poppies. Bromelain, an anti-inflammatory, is derived from pineapple; methyl salicylate from winter greens; quinidine (from the cinchona tree) relieves malaria; aspirin comes from willow bark; and there are many more, too numerous to mention (Veeresham 2012). And did you know that German doctors prescribe herbal remedies as well as conventional medicines? How very sensible! Herbal remedies don't have the severe side effects of some pharmaceutical drugs, and this is why German doctors champion them.

To ridicule herbal remedies is to accuse Mother Nature of quackery! What's heartening is that there's plenty of anecdotal evidence in the form of personal success stories like mine – for example, the story of a Russian soldier who discovered the health benefits of the herb rhodiola (Johnson 2016).

Some of my favourite therapies which I believe are the most helpful in relieving gut and brain symptoms and reducing stress levels are reflexology, aromatherapy massage and acupuncture. There have been several scientific studies showing that acupuncture helps ease IBS, pain, anxiety and depression (Manheimer et al 2012; Rafiei et al 2014). As such, it is now available on the NHS.

Hypnosis

In the past few years, the NHS has studied the effect of hypnotherapy for irritable bowel syndrome with positive results. The beneficial effects appear to last at least five years! (Gonsalkorale et al 2003). Hypnotherapy is an altered state of consciousness like deep relaxation. When you're in this subconscious state, your mind is open to positive suggestions. I don't like the word 'hypnotherapy' because it conjures up pictures of being in a trance-like state, scaring people into believing they would be out of control of their bodies and minds. I've been hypnotised, and this is not the case. I think a more suitable name might be 'positive imagery' or 'positive relaxation', as it involves being talked through positive and helpful images and scenarios while in a relaxed state. It's nothing to fear and can help with many other problems besides IBS.

Emotional Freedom Technique

Emotional freedom technique (EFT) can be used to treat depression, anxiety and pain (Blacher 2023). War veterans with post-traumatic stress disorder have had particularly great results. It's a simple method you can use at home. There are several acupressure points on the body that you tap while vocalising your negative feelings. I had almost miraculous results using EFT during a particularly bad patch of insomnia. I've recommended it to clients, mainly for anxiety, and some of them had equally great results. Brad Yates has some helpful YouTube tutorials (see Resources). I recommend you look him up.

Colonic irrigation

The first recorded account of colonic irrigation was in Egypt around 1500 BC. The forefather of modern medicine, Hippocrates, believed in its health benefits. It has stood the test of time and is still popular today. Colonic irrigation can be a wonderful start to the three-point plan because it empties the bowel and speeds up detoxification and digestive cleansing, relieving pain, constipation and diarrhoea (Hsu et al 2016). Colonic irrigation is a bit like an internal bath. The water gently flows in and out, taking years' worth of poop with it. It massages the bowel wall and encourages proper peristalsis. It's not painful or embarrassing, and you'll feel great afterwards – energised, bright eyed and bushy tailed!

Summing up

I hope some parts of this section have spoken to you, and you've taken a few things from it that you feel you can incorporate into your everyday life to help you manage stress and maintain a feeling of wellbeing. Life can be challenging, so we all need a few tricks up our sleeves to help us manage stress and look after our emotional health. Whichever of the lifestyle options you choose, practise it regularly until it becomes a habit and as natural to you as sleeping or showering. Pop it in your diary, like you would an appointment, to help you commit. Find what works for you and stick with it. We all need something to help keep us sane in this crazy world!

Chapter 11

Point 3: Nutritional supplements

Healthy supplementation

To supplement or not to supplement, that is the question! A dietary supplement is a nutritional product in the form of a capsule, tablet, liquid or powder. It's designed to provide nutrients such as vitamins and minerals, correct deficiencies and support your body to be well. There's a clue in the name 'supplement'. Nutritional supplements are there to *enhance* your diet, not as a substitute for healthy foods.

The reason diet is number one in my three-point plan is because it is the best way to improve your overall health. Supplements are secondary. If your diet is rubbish, all the supplements in the world won't help you feel better. However, diet alone isn't usually enough to reverse deficiencies. Depending on the severity of the deficiency, a short course of supplements may be enough to correct an imbalance, but severe or inherited deficiencies may result in supplementation for life.

Humans are dependent on around 45 nutrients. Every organ, including your brain, requires an adequate supply of vitamins and minerals. They are the raw materials your body needs to function and are essential to health (Tardy et al 2020). The Western diet is lacking in nutrients. High food consumption coupled with low nutrient intake is known as 'hidden hunger' and has reached epidemic levels (Bush & Welsh 2015). Because we have an abundance of food, malnutrition has become overlooked. But most of my clients who have had blood tests to check their vitamin and mineral levels find they are deficient in more than one.

The negative impact of a deficiency in even one vitamin can't be underestimated because each of them is involved in many bodily functions. People with gut dysbiosis have a higher risk of deficiency because vitamin production is an important function of the gut microbiome (Yang et al 2024; Brauer-Nikonow & Zimmermann 2022).

In my opinion, the only way to ensure an adequate supply of vitamins and minerals these days is by taking supplements. This is backed up by a study into the prevalence of inadequate nutrient intake in Europe (Roman Viñas et al 2011). I think there are many factors contributing to the widespread problem of nutritional deficiency. Depletion of minerals from the soil and, therefore, the food grown in that soil is an important factor. So, even if you're eating a balanced diet, the nutrients you expect to be present aren't always there (Thomas 2007).

The planet's microbiome is intimately connected to the human microbiome; they have evolved together. As the soil, water and air become more polluted, so too does the human microbiome. Vegetables and fruit are the most nutritious foods, but because they have been grown in depleted soils and likely sprayed with pesticides, you probably need to eat a lot more fruit and veg than your grandparents would have had to eat to obtain the same nutritional value. A US study found that the nutrient content of vegetables is decreasing and is currently up to 38 per cent lower than in the middle of the 20th century (Lovell n.d.).

Foods are not created equal! The vitamin content in food varies enormously. One study of the selenium content in Brazil nuts showed a 34-fold variation (Silva et al 2017)! Some nuts contained only 2 mg/kg of selenium, while some nuts contained up to 68 mg/

kg. I've heard it said time and time again that there's no need to take supplements if you eat a 'balanced diet'. But it's a nonsensical thing to say because none of us know the exact vitamin content of the food we're eating, although the taste can be a good indicator. I think supermarket vegetables are pretty tasteless compared to the organic veg and salad I grow in my own garden.

Prescription medications that deplete the body

A few examples of commonly used drugs that deplete the body of vitamins are metformin (a popular diabetes drug) and PPIs (prescribed for indigestion), which deplete B vitamins. Statins (prescribed to reduce cholesterol) deplete CoQ10. It has been suggested that this is what causes aches and pains in many people who take statins (Qiao et al 2013). ACE inhibitors (prescribed for high blood pressure) deplete zinc, while SSRIs (prescribed for depression) lower the thyroid hormone (Chong et al 2021).

When should you implement a supplement regime?

In the case of gut dysbiosis, when the gut is likely inflamed and sensitive, supplements might cause further irritation, so it's important to first remove any offending foods and let the gut calm down and start to heal. Your body wants to be well and it continually strives to heal and repair itself, so when you remove the foods that upset your microbiome and replace them with healing, nutritious foods, your gut will quickly start repairing and resume efficient digestion and absorption. You'll be amazed at how quickly your digestive symptoms reduce. Within a few weeks of removing the foods you're sensitive to, your gut function should improve. This is the time to start taking supplements. If you supplement before this point, it's likely you won't be digesting and absorbing them properly, so it's pointless. Nutritional supplements can be quite pricey, so you want to ensure you're getting your money's worth! The good news is that the gut heals and regenerates quickly, so a six-month intensive course of supplements alongside diet and lifestyle changes can result in transformative healing. Then you could go on to a low-maintenance programme.

In this book, I discuss nutritional supplements but not herbal or homoeopathic remedies. This is because I'm not a trained herbalist, but I have a great deal of faith in their efficacy. Here in the UK, herbal remedies are treated with suspicion, but I'm not sure why. Plants and humans have evolved together, and I believe Mother Nature always knows best. For example, St John's wort has been shown to be as effective as conventional antidepressants, with only a fraction of their side effects (Ernst 2000).

Other countries have researched herbal remedies more thoroughly and incorporate them alongside conventional treatments. Cancer care centres in Europe treat patients with extracts from white berry mistletoe (National Cancer Institute n.d.). Mistletoe is nature's original immunotherapy. A Chinese scientific study in 2021 reported more than 90 per cent efficacy of traditional Chinese herbal medicine in relieving lung congestion of patients hospitalised with Covid-19 (Lee et al). Anything that occurs naturally, such as vitamins and minerals, can't be patented, which means there's not much money to be made from them. I think this is the reason why there has been very little research into herbal medicine or foods as medicine – and not because it's quackery, because it most certainly isn't! As a wise person once said, 'Absence of evidence is not evidence of absence.'

The most common side effects I see from taking supplements are mild and include things such as tummy ache, wind, bloating and diarrhoea. This is normal and the symptoms pass as the body adapts. Just lower the dosage or take them every other day for a while. I tend to start my clients on a low dose and build up gradually. Other side effects may occur if you're taking prescribed medication and the supplement interacts with it. For this reason, I recommend you let your GP know which supplements you're planning on taking. Also, please don't stop taking any prescribed medications without the guidance of your doctor.

There's a nutrient level we can survive on, and this is the level on which 'recommended daily allowances' are based. But there's another level for optimum health, and this is the level I try to achieve for my clients. We're all different and our needs vary, and this is why recommended daily allowances (RDAs) aren't very reliable. The RDA for vitamin B3 is 16 mg. But this is the minimum amount needed in a healthy person to avoid deficiency. I believe someone suffering with gut dysbiosis and brain symptoms would likely benefit from around 2,000 mg a day. And it would be impossible to achieve that amount from diet alone. It's not about taking huge amounts of supplements; it's about taking the right amount for you to experience excellent mental and physical health, and this amount will vary from person to person (Munro 1977).

Orthomolecular medicine and brain symptoms

Orthomolecular medicine searches for vitamin and mineral deficiencies as the cause of mental and physical illness. The brain is dependent on adequate nutrition, and vitamin and mineral deficiencies can directly cause brain symptoms.

Orthomolecular psychiatry discovers which vitamins and minerals the patient is deficient in and then finds the optimum doses of those vitamins required by the patient to feel well and symptom free. The fathers of orthomolecular psychiatry are Abram Hoffer and Humphrey Osmond. They had long and successful careers helping schizophrenic patients using high doses of vitamin B3 (Carter 2019). They restored the health of thousands of mentally ill people. I recommend you read some of their inspiring books, which are full of uplifting, real-life stories of people who had been written off by modern medicine or dosed up to their eyeballs on tranquillisers who had their health restored when Hoffer corrected their nutritional deficiencies. He believed that many of his patients who had been diagnosed schizophrenic or psychotic had subclinical pellagra (Hoffer 2008).

Pellagra is a vitamin B3 deficiency and it used to kill thousands of people a year. These days people rarely die of it but even a slight deficiency of B3 can cause gut and brain symptoms (Gasperi et al

2019). Hoffer proved that, in the case of some deficiencies, the sufferer becomes 'vitamin dependent', meaning they must take supplements for the rest of their life. This is true in my case. If I want to stay free from the symptoms of pyrrole disorder and copper overload, I'll have to take B6 and zinc for the rest of my life.

Just because we no longer see cases of scurvy, pellagra and rickets, we wrongly assume we have eradicated the problem of deficiency-related disease but we're a nation of overfed and under-nourished individuals, so it's inevitable that mild vitamin and mineral deficiencies are still causing serious health problems today (Venturelli et al 2021).

We tend to accept fatigue and anxiety and digestive troubles as normal and part of the process of getting old. But it's not normal and it doesn't have to be that way. If we have the appropriate levels of vitamins and minerals to allow all our bodily functions to work correctly, we should feel energised, well and happy. This is the norm but unfortunately most of us have forgotten what that feels like! Vitamins and minerals help you achieve optimum physical and mental health naturally. Vitamins and minerals are not the same as pharmaceutical drugs. They are foods! They can't be put in the same category as antidepressants because they don't disrupt body chemistry; they work *with* body chemistry.

Side effects from nutrients are typically mild. Overdoses are tricky because in general a gigantic amount would have to be taken before it became toxic.

Freud's treatment of mental illness through psychoanalysis has dominated the approach to mental health for over 100 years but a purely psychological hypothesis of mental illness is failing many people and I think a biochemical hypothesis needs more research. I can't stress how valuable an orthomolecular approach to mental and physical health is. However, an orthomolecular approach to mental illness doesn't fit the traditional paradigm, which favours a pharma-ceutical approach, so I fear change will be a long time coming. But I hope I've convinced you that the orthomolecular approach is worth exploring. It can be combined with most standard therapy.

The history of orthomolecular medicine

William J Walsh, Carl C Pfeiffer, Abram Hoffer and Linus Pauling are all doctors and scientists who have researched and proved the efficacy of orthomolecular medicine. Between them they have successfully treated the brain symptoms of thousands of patients. They have analysed millions of blood and urine samples in patients suffering with autism, ADD, clinical depression, anxiety, bipolar syndrome and schizophrenia. Their results show clear trends in chemical imbalances in mentally ill patients that differ from healthy patients – all of which can be corrected with nutrients, with no need for psychiatric medication. Findings on this scale are hardly likely to be coincidence. A few examples of their findings include B6 and zinc deficiency in depressed, anxious patients and niacin deficiency in schizophrenia (Miller & Dulay 2008), copper/zinc imbalance in autism and the trend of copper overload in post-partum depression and other mental illnesses.

Brain science is continually identifying the molecular biology behind more and more mental illnesses. These findings are a revelation because they reveal the causes of mental illness, all of which can be treated nutritionally with no need for psychiatric medication, and yet they fail to become public knowledge. There have been various attempts over the years to discredit these findings but comparatively few attempts to verify them. If these same people who put so much time and money into discrediting an orthomolecular approach genuinely cared about people's health, surely they would set up double-blind, randomised controlled trials that would prove or disprove once and for all the effectiveness of an orthomolecular approach to mental illness? Interestingly, few such studies have been forthcoming.

I've noticed a few trends in my own practice. Most of my clients who test their vitamin and mineral status have a deficiency in zinc and vitamin D, so this is why I always include them as part of my clients' supplement regimen. Another common deficiency I see is one or more of the B vitamins. The other trend, as I've previously mentioned, is that many of my clients with brain symptoms also have digestive problems, so this is why I always recommend a probiotic as part of my supplement regimen. All these clients who then followed my three-point plan and retested after six months saw an improvement in their test results and the majority were no longer classed as deficient.

Last but not least, since the Covid-19 pandemic, there has been a huge increase in depression and brain symptoms. One study showed a seven-fold increase (Bueno-Notivol et al 2021)! This puts a huge burden on healthcare services, making a non-prescription, nutrient approach even more valuable.

Case study

I recently met a 15-year-old client with brain symptoms. She was highly anxious and depressed; she'd stopped socialising and was missing a lot of school days. Her diet wasn't great by my standards, but typical by Western standards. She had been a strict vegetarian between the ages of 12 and 14. My practice is small, so this may just be coincidence, but I've seen this link between vegetarianism and brain symptoms in a few of my young clients, and I suspect that because the teenage body has a high demand for nutrients, some teenagers who try vegetarianism may become deficient.

Her parents were keen for her to avoid prescription medicine and were open to my suggestion of blood tests to check for vitamin and mineral deficiency. They went to their GP, who checked her vitamin D and B12 status. The results revealed that she was deficient in both. And so she began a supplement programme: 3,000 IU vitamin D3 daily and also a course of B12 injections.

The transformation in her emotional wellbeing was miraculous! It would be normal for a supplement programme to take three months or more before improvements were noticeable, but this young woman was feeling bright eyed, bushy tailed and almost back to her usual self within a month, which was wonderful.

PS: Other clients who were vitamin deficient have seen great improvement after supplementation. But I must admit the results are usually slower to achieve.

Many people in the UK are deficient in vitamin D because of our diabolical weather! A lack of sunshine, especially in the autumn and winter months can lead to deficiency and so I believe everyone living in the UK should supplement during the winter months. A deficiency in vitamin D is associated with depression (Anglin et al 2013). This has been the case for many, many years, but it's only recently that GPs have regularly started testing for and prescribing vitamin D. In the future, I'd like to see them testing the full range of vitamins and minerals. I just wish that more money went into researching the cause of illness. Imagine if we all regularly had our vitamin and mineral status checked for free at the GP's surgery. It would help us stay in tip-top health. I believe the only thing that could be considered a drawback to an orthomolecular approach is that nutrients can take a few months to take effect, whereas psychiatric medications can kick in very quickly.

Improvements in gut health usually occur quite quickly when following my three-point plan, probably because I remove a lot of the gut irritants. However, improvements in brain symptoms often take a little longer – months rather than weeks. It also takes months to correct vitamin and mineral deficiencies.

I have listed below the supplements I find benefit most of my gut and brain clients. I don't recommend you take all of them at once! I've purposefully omitted dosage because the amount varies according to the individual's needs. I'd prefer you to work with a nutritionist who can guide you through an in-depth questionnaire that will indicate which vitamins and minerals you lack and what dosage you should take. But if you want to be sure, there are blood tests available that will let you know exactly which vitamins and minerals you are deficient in. In my experience the results almost always come back showing deficiency in several.

Most of my clients can't afford expensive testing, but they get great results from following my diet recommendations and taking a few of the nutritional supplements I consider to be essential. Studies have shown that people who take supplements are healthier and at a lower risk of disease than non-supplement takers (Block et al 2007).

I have listed the supplements in order of importance, starting with the ones I consider to be essential for clients suffering with gut and brain symptoms. I've followed this up with a list of optional supplements.

The supplements I commonly recommend

See also the Resources section for a full list of suggested suppliers at the time of writing.

Berberine

What it is: Berberine is one of the most powerful plant remedies available and has been shown to be as effective as some pharmaceutical drugs (Berry 2023). It can be extracted from several different plants and is classed as an alkaloid. An alkaloid is a naturally occurring compound of plant origin that has a profound physiological effect on humans. To put this into context, I'll give you a few examples of other powerful alkaloids: caffeine found in coffee, morphine (which comes from the poppy plant), quinine (the malaria drug, which comes from the bark of the cinchona tree) and belladonna (which is probably best known for being a poison and used today in small amounts in prescription-only antispasmodic medication). Never underestimate the power of plants!

What it's good for: Most importantly, in the case of gut dysbiosis, it's antimicrobial – meaning it helps to keep your gut microbes in balance. It's antifungal and therefore works against *Candida* overgrowth (Xie et al 2020). It also improves the number of short-chain fatty acids in the gut, reducing inflammation and strengthening the intestinal barrier, which helps to heal a leaky gut. It also helps small intestinal bacterial overgrowth (SIBO), relaxes painful gut spasms and eases diarrhoea and bacterial gastroenteritis. It also supports the liver in detoxification, so it really is a magic remedy for the gut. It also increases serotonin and dopamine, meaning that it helps depression (Zhan et al 2021). It's also a cancer cell inhibitor (Almatroodi et al

2022), boosts immunity and lowers blood pressure. It promotes fat metabolism and so may be helpful for weight loss. It's also antiviral, antiparasitic and anti-inflammatory (Ye et al 2021).

Berberine is known as 'nature's metformin', which is a drug used to treat type 2 diabetes. It's so effective at controlling blood glucose that some diabetics have been able to come off their medication. Berberine is effective in treating infections, and it has helped some clients to avoid antibiotics. All of these wonderful benefits come from one simple plant remedy. How clever Mother Nature is! She offers us solutions to many of our maladies (Och et al 2022).

You're probably scratching your head and asking why you've never heard of berberine before. That's because it's a relatively new remedy in the UK. However, the Chinese have been using it for hundreds of years. But they are much more knowledgeable than us when it comes to plant and herbal remedies. There's talk of berberine becoming a prescription-only drug in the UK. I hope this doesn't happen because it will massively restrict its use, and it seems unnecessary because it's extremely safe. The majority of people I recommend berberine to feel the benefits. And so, over the years, it's become a firm favourite of mine.

Side effects: Until the body gets used to it, berberine can temporarily upset sensitive tummies. If this happens, just lower your dosage.

Cautions: It may interact with medication that lowers blood sugar. Use with caution if you have low blood pressure. Don't use if you're pregnant or nursing.

My preferred supplement: I recommend Clean Berberine by British Supplements (british-supplements.net).

Berberine is expelled from the body within a few hours. So, for this reason, I recommend you spread out your intake over three separate doses. I recommend taking it with your main meals to take advantage of its positive effect on blood sugar.

Vitamin C

What it is: The more I read about Vitamin C, the more I champion it and recommend it to just about everyone for just about everything! It strengthens the immune system and fights infections. It produces collagen, keeping your bones strong and your skin young. It's an antioxidant, an antihistamine, helps to make anti-stress hormones and turns food into energy. But most important are its positive effects on the gut (Otten et al 2021). It promotes healthy bacteria, which helps to correct gut dysbiosis. And it's also a powerful antimicrobial, which kills off the bacteria and yeasts fermenting in your gut. The stomach is supposed to be a sterile place, and vitamin C sterilises the upper gut, helping to fight against small intestine bacterial overgrowth (Deruelle & Baron 2008). Sugar and stress lead to vitamin C deficiency, so I'd like to bet the majority of Westerners are deficient. The best food sources are fruit, vegetables and parsley. Most species make their own vitamin C, but humans do not. Therefore it's extremely important that we obtain Vitamin C daily from food and supplements. It's doubtful we can obtain enough from diet alone, so it's one of the few supplements I always recommend.

Side effects: Diarrhoea is the most common side effect. For this reason, start your dosage low and slowly work up to bowel tolerance level.

Cautions: It may not be suitable if you have a blood disorder or kidney stones.

My preferred supplement: Holfords Immune C available in tablet or powder form. It also contains antioxidants and zinc.

Dosage: As I mentioned earlier dosages vary from person to person. But for the maximum benefit it's important you take vitamin C to bowel tolerance level.

Anywhere between 1 and 10 grams a day is a safe dose. Start off with 1 gram taken in the morning and 1 gram taken last thing at night. Keep increasing this dose every few days until you find your bowel tolerance level. By this, I mean until you get the squits! Once you've worked out the amount for your own personal bowel tolerance, drop the dose slightly so it no longer upsets your tummy. Vitamin C can't be stored in the body for more than about six hours, so this is the reason I recommend you take it morning and night – but most importantly, last thing at night on an empty stomach. This allows the vitamin C to sterilise your upper gut and kill any bad bacteria while you sleep.

Digestive enzymes

What they do: Digestive enzymes are released by your body every time you eat. They help you to digest fats, carbohydrates and proteins (Ianiro et al 2016). But various things deplete the body's supply of enzymes, such as a deficiency in zinc, old age and digestive troubles. An ample supply of digestive enzymes is essential for you to digest your food. I've seen a lot of clients find relief from their gut symptoms after introducing a digestive enzyme. If you suffer from regular indigestion, diarrhoea and food sensitivities, you'll likely benefit from supplementing (Spagnuolo et al 2017). As you follow the three-point plan and your digestion and vitamin status improve, you may no longer need to take digestive enzymes.

Best food sources: Enzymes are naturally present in raw food, but cooking destroys them – another reason not to overcook your veg! Sauerkraut is a great source of digestive enzymes (see Recipes), so if you prefer, rather than taking a digestive enzyme, you could just have a couple of mouthfuls of sauerkraut before your meal.

Side effects: They may irritate ulcerative conditions of the gut and cause slight heartburn.

Cautions: Don't take if you're pregnant or breastfeeding.

My preferred supplement: I like Solgar's Chewable Vegan Digestive Enzymes because I'm not very good at swallowing tablets and capsules.

Betaine hydrochloride

What it does: Hydrochloric acid (HCl) is a fancy name for stomach acid. Stomach acid has many essential functions. It digests your food, sterilises your upper gut and is part of your immune defence against microbes, yeast and harmful bacteria (Levy 2023). In addition, optimal stomach acid levels are essential to absorb vitamins and minerals from your food. A lack of stomach acid leads to a condition called small intestine bacterial overgrowth (SIBO), which we discussed in an earlier chapter.

Age, stress and a deficiency in B6 and zinc can all contribute to a depletion in your levels of stomach acid. If indigestion and reflux is a common problem for you, you may benefit from supplementing HCl (Kines & Krupczak 2016). Apple cider vinegar can increase stomach acid levels and it's a cheaper option than supplements. A couple of tablespoons with your main meals should do the trick. Freshly squeezed lemon juice also stimulates the production of HCl. Undigested food in your poop is a sign that you need to supplement HCl and digestive enzymes.

Side effects: Heartburn is really the only side effect so start on a low dose and work up.

Cautions: Don't take if you have peptic ulcers, are pregnant or are breastfeeding.

My preferred supplement: Nutri Advanced sell a great supplement called Nutrigest. This contains all the digestive enzymes we just discussed above, plus betaine HCl.

L-glutamine

What it does: L-glutamine is an amino acid that has a positive healing effect on both gut and brain symptoms (Zhou et al 2019). It helps to heal a leaky gut and prevents bacteria and toxins moving from your intestines into the rest of your body (Dos Santos et al 2010). It's anti-inflammatory and reduces the inflammation associated with acid reflux. It also helps to control food cravings and benefits people with food sensitivities. L-glutamine plays an important role in strengthening immunity and is a powerful antioxidant. It's produced in your body, but if you have gut dysbiosis, you'll almost certainly need more than your body can produce, so you'll benefit from supplementing. L-glutamine also benefits mental health. It's known as the calming amino acid because it's a substrate (underlying substance) for the neurotransmitter GABA and helps to reduce anxiety and depression (Son et al 2018).

Best food sources: Meat and animal products such as eggs and beef are the best source.

Side effects: Because glutamine is naturally produced in the body, using the supplement is considered safe.

Cautions: People with kidney disease, liver disease, cancer, Reye's syndrome, or anyone taking medication for seizures may need to avoid taking L-glutamine, as should pregnant and breastfeeding women. Don't exceed doses of 30 grams daily.

My preferred supplement: BioCares' L-Glutamine Powder. It's best taken on an empty stomach, so I recommend first thing on a morning or last thing at night, or both.

Probiotics

What they do: The word probiotic has Latin and Greek origins and translates to 'for life'. Probiotics are a type of friendly bacteria that live in your gut. They can also be taken in supplement form to replenish and support your gut microbiome. Your microbiome is full of good and bad bacteria, and taking a probiotic supplement gives bad bacteria less chance of survival. It's possible to get probiotics from food sources, but if you have gut dysbiosis, I think you'll need the additional support of supplements for a few months. Probiotics have a wide range of health benefits: they correct gut dysbiosis, reduce inflammation, aid weight loss, reduce depression and anxiety, reduce symptoms of irritable bowel syndrome, treat infections, reduce acne, lower cholesterol, boost immune function, manufacture B vitamins, improve heart health, calm allergic reactions and redress the balance of the gut microbiome (Brown 2023).

If your digestive symptoms started after taking antibiotics, then probiotics are essential for your recovery. If you ever need to take a course of antibiotics in the future, I recommend you take probiotics, vitamin C and L-glutamine during and after the course. And follow a low-carbohydrate diet because antibiotics cause bad microbes to proliferate and carbohydrates feed them.

Best food sources: Probiotic foods include fermented foods such as yoghurt, kefir, sauerkraut, miso, kimchi, tempeh and pickles. I'm a big fan of fermented foods because they're healing and nourishing for the gut.

Side effects: Wind, bloating and diarrhoea – these are all symptoms of the positive changes taking place in the gut microbiota. The good bacteria proliferate and the bad bacteria die off. This may cause some mild effects known as the 'die-off reaction'. Symptoms include headache, nausea and an upset tummy. The good news is that this is only short lived and usually mild. If you experience any side effects from probiotic supplementation, take a day or two off and start again on a very small dose and slowly build up. Take a probiotic supplement for at least three to six months. You must stick to a healthy diet during this time. Processed foods, alcohol and sugar will negate the positive effects of probiotic supplements.

Cautions: People with HIV have been known to develop infections while taking probiotics.

My preferred supplements: Symprove is one of my favourites because the good bacteria it contains have been proven to survive the journey through the gut, meaning a good supply of live probiotics is delivered where it's needed. Plus, it's gluten-free and tastes yummy!

Another of my favourites is Bio Acidophilus Forte, by BioCare. There are many different strains of probiotics, but the two main ingredients used in this supplement are lactobacilli and bifidobacteria. In scientific studies, these two strains have been shown to be low in the guts of people with gut and brain symptoms (Aizawa et al 2016). They strengthen the gut lining and reduce inflammatory reactions to food and have been shown to reduce depression and anxiety in countless other studies.

Another source of probiotic is a supplement called Lepicol. It was designed by a chap who couldn't find relief from his IBS symptoms. It's a wonderful source of gentle fibre and is ideal for long-term use. So, if you feel you aren't getting enough fibre from your diet, Lepicol could be the answer. In addition, it regulates bowel movements, meaning it's beneficial for both constipation and diarrhoea.

Another of my favourite supplements is a *prebiotic* called glucomannan, derived from the konjac plant. Prebiotics are foods that we can't digest but our gut microbes can, so think of them as food for your gut microbiome. When you put glucomannan powder in water it swells to several times its size, encouraging peristalsis and regular bowel movements.

Essential fatty acids

What they do: As their name suggests, these polyunsaturated fats are essential to human health. Our ancestors evolved eating marine foods and they are just as essential to our development and health today. There are two families of essential fatty acids: omega 3 and omega 6. The body can't make them from scratch, so they must be obtained from foods. They're important for brain health and the absorption of vitamins and minerals. They help produce hormones, promote bacterial diversity in the gut, improve insulin resistance, reduce risk of heart attack, reduce anxiety and stimulate bile production.

Studies have shown that omega 3 is effective in reducing depression (Grosso et al 2014). This is possibly because depression is an inflammatory condition and omega 3 reduces inflammation. I recommend Basant Puri's book, *The Natural Way To Beat Depression* (2005). He has reported a 100 per cent success rate in treating depressed patients with an omega 3 fatty acid.

Omega 3 is anti-inflammatory and omega 6 is pro-inflammatory. For this reason, it's important not to consume excessive amounts of omega 6 (Gunnars 2023). There's some concern that the Western diet contains too much omega 6, which is contributing towards inflammatory diseases. I recommend you eat fewer refined seed oils such as vegetable oils, safflower oil, soybean oil, canola oil, sunflower oil, sesame oil, rice bran oil and peanut oil, all of which are found in processed foods.

Best food sources of omega 3: Oily fish, leafy green vegetables, algae, linseeds, chia seeds, walnuts, grass-fed meat, omega 3-enriched eggs.

Side effects: Belching, nausea, loose stools.

Cautions: Don't use fish oils for cooking. I recommend cooking with lard or coconut oil. Fish oils may thin the blood, so they aren't advisable to take alongside warfarin or aspirin.

My preferred supplement: Mega EPA Forte by BioCare.

Zinc

What it does: You may have noticed that a zinc deficiency is present in many of the conditions I've mentioned. It's very common in people diagnosed with mental illness (Grønli et al 2013).

This has certainly been the case in my own practice. Many of my clients who have tested their zinc status have been deficient, and every one of them has seen an improvement in brain symptoms when they include a zinc supplement as part of their regimen. Zinc is required for the regulation of GABA, the calming neurotransmitter. It plays a part in the production of digestive enzymes and stomach acid, heals and repairs the gut wall, reduces fermenting in the gut and gut inflammation, aids the ability to deal with stress and boosts immunity. I recommend you take more zinc during stressful times (Kubala 2022).

Signs of zinc deficiency: Diarrhoea, white spots on nails, mouth ulcers, hair loss, weak immune system, anxiety, impotence, loss of appetite, blurred vision, brain fog, low insulin and poor blood sugar control.

Interesting titbit

The symptoms of zinc deficiency are very similar to the symptoms of anorexia nervosa. There are studies showing that people with eating disorders are zinc deficient and have made a good recovery after supplementing with zinc (Greenblatt 2021).

Best food sources: Red meat, shellfish, fresh root ginger, pecans, almonds, seeds, eggs, dark chocolate.

Side effects: Stomach irritation, metallic taste in the mouth.

Cautions: Zinc can cause nausea if taken too early in the day or on an empty stomach. It's important to increase zinc intake gradually because it can cause an overload of toxic metals and copper as they're expelled from the body; 90 mg a day is considered a safe dose, but I always start people on 15 mg a day and work up slowly.

Zinc can block the absorption of iron and manganese. So if my clients take zinc long term I recommend they take Floradix liquid iron and BioCares liquid manganese.

My preferred supplement: Zinc works best when it's taken alongside B6 and magnesium. Last thing at night is the best time to treat a fermenting gut. I recommend Zinc 30 by Pure Encapsulations.

An easy, cheap test to see if you're deficient in zinc is the 'taste test'. I use Lambert's Zincatest. It's a liquid zinc solution that can be used as a supplement and also as an indicator of your zinc status. Simply swirl the solution around your mouth for ten seconds. If you can't taste anything it indicates you are zinc deficient.

Vitamin D

What it does: In scientific studies, supplementation with vitamin D has been shown to improve the symptoms associated with irritable bowel syndrome and it plays an important role in the integrity of the intestinal lining (Jalili et al 2019). This is why it's one of my favourite supplements because of its healing effect on the gut. Studies show it restores the tight junctions of the intestine wall, thereby repairing a leaky gut (Lee et al 2019). It's also anti-inflammatory and is essential for a healthy immune system. In addition, vitamin D3 enhances calcium and magnesium absorption and helps deposit them in the bones. It's therefore one of the best preventative supplements to help protect against osteoporosis. A deficiency in vitamin D is a common cause of depression (Shipowick et al 2009), so I think it might be helpful if GPs tested their patients' vitamin D status before prescribing antidepressants. Ideally you want a blood level above 100 nmol/l and certainly no lower than 70 nmol/l. To achieve these levels, try to get at least half an hour of sun exposure daily. But during the winter there isn't sufficient sunshine, so I recommend everyone supplements. Signs of vitamin

D deficiency include fatigue, insomnia, aches and pains, poor immunity, hair loss, weight gain and anxiety.

Best food sources: Fish, eggs, red meat, liver.

Cautions: Excessive intake can lead to soft tissue calcification, but this would take levels far exceeding any recommended dosage. Don't exceed 3000 IU a day.

My preferred supplement: I like BioCare's liquid D3 and K2. D3 and K2 work synergistically to support bone health.

Sometimes vitamin D is expressed in terms of international units (IU) and sometimes as micrograms (mcg) Just to confuse things further, the word microgram is sometimes written with Greek symbols (µg). One microgram (or µg) of vitamin D is equivalent to 40 IU.

Vitamin B6

What it does: B6 is essential for digestion because it's necessary for the formation of stomach acid and digestive enzymes. People with B6 deficiency tend towards depression because it's necessary for the synthesis of serotonin and GABA. And so, B6 supplementation works as a natural antidepressant. It also helps to control allergic reactions and reduce inflammation (Kennedy 2016). A deficiency causes gut and brain symptoms, sleep disorders, irritability, poor immunity, dermatitis, cracked corners of the mouth, sore tongue, fatigue and tingling in the hands and feet. You may have noticed that B6 deficiency is seen in some of the conditions I've mentioned: pyrrole disorder and copper overload. B6 deficiency is often genetic, meaning supplementation will probably be lifelong. B6 is one of the more common deficiencies I've seen over the years. However, I should point out that all of the B vitamins play an important role in healthy brain function.

Best food sources: Seeds, nuts, Brussels sprouts, watercress, cauliflower, cabbage, broccoli, asparagus.

Side effects: Some people may experience nausea or tummy ache. High doses may cause nightmares and/or peripheral neuropathy (numbness or tingling in the hands and feet). Lowering the dose will solve this.

Cautions: There's no known toxicity if you follow the recommended dosage. It can disrupt sleep, so don't take in the evening or exceed 200mg daily.

My preferred supplement: I usually recommend P5P, the active form of B6. I like Pure Encapsulations' P5P. B vitamins are water soluble and any excess is excreted from the body in the urine.

In my experience, B6 is one of the lesser-tolerated supplements. I've seen it trigger upset tummy and nausea in quite a few people. This could be because some B6 supplements contain yeast, and I suspect many of my patients with gut dysbiosis have some degree of *Candida* overgrowth. Just start on a very low dose and build up slowly.

Magnesium

What it does: Magnesium aids restful sleep, eases anxiety (Boyle et al 2017), relaxes muscles and helps to ease painful spasms in the gut. It also relieves constipation, calms excess stomach acid and eases migraines. Magnesium deficiency is extremely common. Magnesium plays an important role in the prevention of osteoporosis.

Best food sources: Almonds, Brazil nuts, garlic, crab, green leafy vegetables.

Side effects: Blushing of the skin, thirst, low blood pressure, diarrhoea.

Cautions: People with kidney disease should avoid supplementing. Don't exceed 1000 mg daily. Magnesium interacts with calcium so if you are taking magnesium long term make sure you have an adequate calcium intake in your diet or take a calcium supplement.
My preferred supplements: MegaMag Muscleze by Nutri Advanced

is great. This combines magnesium glycinate (which is calming and benefits insomnia), calcium and B6. However, it also contains folic acid, which doesn't suit everyone. I also like Magnesium Taurate, made by Viridian. It contains the amino acid taurine, which is calming and anti-inflammatory.

Interesting titbit

Over the past 15 years, I've recommended 300 mg of magnesium before bed to hundreds of people with sleep problems and I estimate more than 50 per cent of them have seen an improvement in the quality of their sleep, so it's definitely worth a try!

Optional supplements

These are supplements I recommend less often, depending on the symptoms my clients are presenting with.

Peppermint capsules

Peppermint reduces bloating and tummy ache. In addition, there are many studies showing that peppermint oil reduces the symptoms of IBS (NHS 2021).

Best food sources: Mint is an easy herb to grow in your garden. You can make your own mint tea by popping a few leaves in a mug and pouring hot water over them.

Side effects: Heartburn, headache, skin flushing.

Cautions: No known contraindications.

My preferred supplement: Peppermint capsules are available over the counter from most pharmacies. I like Colpermin IBS Relief Capsules.

5-HTP

This is a great natural alternative to antidepressants. You've probably heard of serotonin, which is sometimes called the happy hormone because it stabilises mood and creates feelings of wellbeing and happiness. 5-HTP is converted into serotonin, which in turn increases melatonin production. Melatonin has many beneficial effects on both gut and brain symptoms. Unfortunately, over-the-counter sales were banned in Europe and it's now a prescription-only medication. Because melatonin is produced by the body, it's extremely safe to supplement, so it's a shame its usage has been restricted. If you feel you'd benefit, it may be worth speaking to your doctor, who can prescribe a melatonin supplement for you. Otherwise, taking 5-HTP will boost melatonin production (Van De Walle 2023). Several clients of mine have used 5-HTP in conjunction with weaning themselves off antidepressants, with successful results.

Best food sources: The amino acid tryptophan, which the body uses to make 5-HTP, is found in turkey, chicken, spinach, bananas, pumpkin seeds, sunflower seeds and seaweed.

Side effects: Heartburn, stomach ache, nausea.

Caution: Don't use when breastfeeding or pregnant. And don't exceed 300 mg daily.

My preferred supplement: Patrick Holford's Mood Food.

B vitamins

The B vitamins are water soluble, so any excess is easily excreted in the urine and they are generally very low in toxicity. I never recommend a B complex supplement to clients experiencing brain symptoms because the majority contain folic acid. William Walsh cautions against taking folic acid without first taking a blood test because it can worsen brain symptoms in some folate types. And for the same reason I rarely recommend a multivitamin to clients with brain symptoms because the majority of multivitamin supplements also contain folic acid. Probably the most common deficiencies I've seen over the years are in B6 and B12. But all the B vitamins are connected to brain health, so I recommend people run tests for all of them.

What they do: B vitamins play an important role in mental health and are effective in treating anxiety and depression. This is probably because many of the B vitamins directly impact the brain and nervous system. For example, one of their roles is to make calming neurotransmitters such as GABA and serotonin. A poor diet high in refined carbohydrates depletes B vitamins, as do stress, the contraceptive pill, gut dysbiosis and autoimmune disorders.

The B vitamins play many important roles. Here are just a few: B1 and biotin have proven effective in treating panic symptoms and anxiety. Choline (formerly known as B4) has a calming effect on the body. B3 is known as 'nature's Valium' because of its calming effect. Folic acid balances female hormones. So, the B vitamins may play an essential part in recovery from brain symptoms (Young et al 2019).

Signs of a deficiency depend on which B vitamins you're deficient in, but they include brain symptoms, fatigue, poor concentration, weakness, heart palpitations, shortness of breath, nerve problems, anaemia, sore tongue, nausea, headache, bright red tongue and cracked lips.

Vitamin B3

I often recommend B3 to clients who describe themselves as nervy because of its sedative effect. B3 has benzodiazepine-like benefits without any of the negative side effects. It calms anxiety, aids the function of the gastrointestinal tract, benefits cerebral allergy, lowers histamine levels, helps insomnia, repairs a leaky gut, boosts brain function, converts food into energy, is an antioxidant and also an antipsychotic (Gasperi et al 2019).

A common biochemical imbalance in people who have panic attacks is an excess of lactic acid. The best way to redress this balance is to practise calm, diaphragmatic breathing. Keep your blood sugar levels stable, and take a B3 supplement. Signs of deficiency include: irritable bowel syndrome, headaches, nervousness, fatigue, depression, insomnia, bright red tongue, suicidal thoughts, paranoia and rough skin that becomes pigmented in the sun.

Interesting titbit
Did you know that B3 (nicotinic acid) is effective in lowering cholesterol levels (Shah et al 2013)?

Best food sources: Liver, salmon, anchovies, pork, peanuts, avocado, mushrooms.

Side effects: Diarrhoea, bloating, headache, low blood pressure, skin flushing, itchy skin, rapid heartbeat.

Cautions: B3 may slow blood clotting. Avoid if taking blood thinners. It may increase blood glucose levels.

My preferred supplement: Patrick Holford's No Blush Niacin. Don't exceed 2,000 mg a day. I recommend separating this into two separate doses.

Vitamin B12
What it is: As with all the other B vitamins, B12 deficiency can cause brain symptoms such as panic attacks, phobias, OCD and anxiety. B12 is involved in the synthesis of serotonin and so a deficiency can also cause depression (WebMD 2023). Other signs of deficiency include pale skin, eye twitching, constipation, diarrhoea, fatigue, palpitations and breathlessness. IBS and B12 deficiency have been linked in sufferers who have bacterial overgrowth in the small intestine and people who have low stomach acid. Gut dysbiosis may put you at higher risk of not getting enough B12 from diet alone. I've seen a B12 deficiency in several of my clients who are vegetarian or vegan. This may be because B12 isn't found in plant foods.

Best food sources: Eggs, yoghurt, liver, beef, salmon.

Side effects: Nausea, upset tummy, headache, fatigue, tingling in the hands and feet.

Cautions: B12 supplements may interact with PPIs. Complications may arise in people with kidney disease. The body only absorbs a small percentage of a B12 supplement and for this reason I think B12 injections are best.

Chromium

What it is: Chromium helps to keep blood sugar levels stable and aids the actions of the hormone insulin (Pei et al 2006). It also reduces depression (Davidson et al 2003) and can reduce hunger cravings and binge eating (Brownley et al 2013). It has been used in the treatment of bipolar disorder and schizophrenia.

Best food sources: Fruits (especially apples and oranges), tomato juice, vegetables (especially green beans), beef, liver, eggs, chicken, oysters, wheatgerm, broccoli.

Side effects: Headache, insomnia, upset tummy, mood changes.

Cautions: It may interact with some medications, so check with your GP before taking, especially if you have liver or kidney problems or anaemia. Don't exceed 300 mcg daily.

My preferred supplement: BioCare Nutrisorb Chromium. Don't exceed 300 mcg a day.

Glutathione

What it is: Glutathione is the master antioxidant. Levels in the body decrease with age, stress, poor diet and exposure to toxins. Supplementing with glutathione helps reduces oxidative stress. I mentioned earlier that oxidative stress is implicated in many mental illnesses, so I regularly recommend glutathione supplementation.

Best food sources: Cruciferous vegetables, eggs, lean protein.

Side effects: Tummy ache, diarrhoea.

Cautions: It may interact with other medications, so check with your GP before taking. Don't exceed 200 mg daily.

My preferred supplement: Liposomal Glutathione by Loveliposomal.

Case study

I decided to include this case study of a 54-year-old female because it's a classic example of one of my clients who couldn't afford blood tests but still got great results.

Symptoms: Alternating constipation and diarrhoea, indigestion, bowel incontinence, hot flushes, brain fog, depression, anger.

Background: My client felt that a combination of a divorce and the menopause was the trigger for her declining health. She felt depressed and began comfort eating junk foods and drinking alcohol every evening as a way of relaxing. She'd been prone to bloating and occasional constipation for as long as she could remember but her gut symptoms suddenly worsened, and she was given a diagnosis of irritable bowel syndrome by her doctor. She tried laxatives, antacids and an antidepressant but stopped all three abruptly after only a few weeks of taking. I think this lack of compliance was because she felt so depressed she couldn't even find the motivation to take the tablets. She carried on comfort eating and drinking for a few more months until she reached a low point after a couple of 'accidents' when she accidentally pooped herself. This was when she decided she needed to take responsibility for her health and make some changes to her diet and lifestyle. And so she booked an appointment with me. She couldn't afford any tests, but an in-depth symptom analysis suggested she had gut dysbiosis and was deficient in zinc. I would have loved her to take a hair mineral analysis because I suspected she had raised levels of toxic minerals. There were a few indicators, including dark circles under her eyes, she was overweight, and she said she felt extreme anger all the time. Anger can be a symptom of menopause, but it can also be an indicator of high levels of lead. Lead accumulates in our bones over a lifetime but as bone density breaks down during the menopause, toxic minerals may be released into the bloodstream. Vitamin C helps to carry toxic minerals out of the body.

Three-point plan

» Dietary changes: Remove the alcohol and sugary processed comfort foods that were irritating her gut and incorporate my food suggestions as laid out in this book.
» Lifestyle change: I recommended she find something therapeutic to do with her evenings to break the pattern of comfort eating and drinking. She started going for a long walk followed by a bath, which took up a couple of hours and made her evenings feel less long and lonely.
» Supplements:

› Berberine to rebalance the gut microbiome. Her gut symptoms suggested she had gut dysbiosis after months of high-sugar foods and alcohol.
› Vitamin C: Again to help rebalance the gut microbiome and reduce the oxidative stress caused by alcohol. Plus, it carries toxic minerals out of the body. Vitamin C is a chelator, meaning it latches on to heavy metals and escorts them out of the body.
› Digestive enzyme and HCl combination: To aid digestion and reduce indigestion.
› Omega 3: To reduce inflammation and depression.

> › Zinc: To heal the gut, help balance hormones and regulate insulin and reduce brain symptoms.
> › Red clover tincture: To help reduce menopausal symptoms. The reason I recommend a tincture is because it can easily be added to drinks several times a day. The trick is to keep the hormone receptor sites covered all day long and so one dose in the morning wouldn't help very much because its effects would only last a few hours,
> › Probiotic: This was incorporated after a month to replenish the gut microbiome.

Follow-up: The improvements in her gut symptoms were almost immediate and she said her digestion was much improved. She initially struggled to comply with my diet recommendations, but this inevitably triggered unpleasant gut symptoms, which motivated her to go back to clean eating. She didn't initially tell me she had psoriasis and I couldn't see it because it was covered by clothes. But at the follow-up she told me it had almost gone. This may be because she cut out gluten, which has been linked to psoriasis (Michaelsson et al 2003).

She estimated a 50 per cent reduction in brain fog and hot flushes, which was probably a combination of the red clover and cutting out alcohol. Her depression had only lifted slightly. She estimated a 30 per cent improvement. I think this is because she had reactive depression as a response to the trauma and grief associated with her divorce. So, I recommended she consult a counsellor who could help her work through this. I kept in touch with her occasionally by text message and her health continued to improve. She still followed a clean diet, but scaled back her supplements to just berberine, vitamin C and red clover. She found a great counsellor who helped her process the emotions from her divorce, but she told me the biggest relief was feeling confident she would never again experience bowel incontinence.

Summing up

What I've discussed in the book thus far could be described as preventative medicine. Preventative healthcare includes preventing disease, halting disease and healing from disease. Diet, environmental factors, nutritional status and lifestyle choices all contribute towards the manifestation of disease. However, all of them are within your control. In my opinion, modern-day medicine, as we all know it, isn't focused on preventative medicine. Pharmaceutical companies have turned health into a money-making business. I'm not disputing that there are some wonderful medicines out there – but why are we all sicker than ever? The incidence of conditions such as cancer and mental illness is steadily rising. I believe it's because our approach to health is completely skew-whiff! People wait to become ill and then expect a pill to fix them. I think the solution is to take preventative medicine seriously and incorporate it into your everyday life.

Interesting titbit

Prescription medications are estimated to be the third leading cause of death in the United States and Europe (Gøtzsche 2014)! Interestingly, side effects from prescription medication are never listed as a cause of death on a death certificate, so the true extent of the problem isn't fully understood. This statistic is just one more reason why I think we should all take a preventative approach to our health.

Start eating a diet that promotes excellent health and ensures you're not deficient in vitamins and minerals. Take supplements when needed. Exercise regularly. Look after your emotional health by mastering meditation, mindfulness or yoga. Have a regular massage or acupuncture treatment. All these things are beneficial to your future health and wellbeing. Instead of waiting until we become sick, we should all be taking responsibility for our own health and wellbeing every day. It should be the norm. This is what preventative medicine is all about.

It's a simple equation: less medication, less sugar, less social media, less alcohol, fewer chemicals, fewer pesticides, fewer processed foods, fewer seed oils, fewer late nights, plus more nutrient-dense foods, more vitamins and minerals, more relaxation, more nurturing, more knowledge and more connection equals a happier, healthier you with a better quality of life.

Since 2020, Alicja Baczynska, a specialist registrar, has been urging UK politicians to overhaul the current healthcare system. She is quoted as saying, 'It is unacceptable that the NHS is collapsing under the weight of chronic disease, the majority of which could be prevented and treated by addressing diet and lifestyle factors.' She is leading other doctors to petition the government to shift the direction of the NHS from treating chronic disease to instead preventing it through diet (WorldHealth.net 2020). We need more people like this brave doctor to stick their heads above the parapet and demand change.

A UK government report that looked at the long-term sustainability of the NHS produced some interesting facts and figures (Parliament 2017). Did you know that in the UK, 89 per cent of deaths are caused by preventable disease? The World Health Organization states that four of the most important risk factors for these diseases are tobacco smoke, physical inactivity, alcohol and unhealthy eating. The UK health forum warned that the burden of preventable disease on the NHS is unsustainable, with obesity costing the NHS around £5.1 billion a year.

The same report touched on mental healthcare stating that mental health problems cause 23 per cent of all illnesses in the UK, but mental health services receive only 11 per cent of health spending. Unfortunately two thirds of people with mental health problems receive no appropriate treatment. The report concludes that the NHS must shift from an 'illness' to a 'wellness' service.

These figures highlight the importance of taking responsibility for our own physical and mental health with diet and nutrition. Putting all those facts and figures into simple terms, it means that the majority of people in hospitals right now could have avoided being ill if only they had taken better care of their health. This is encouraging and empowering information, and it puts your health in your hands. What you do with it is your choice.

The low-fat lie

I wonder how many diseases would be prevented if people ate a nutritious diet. But processed foods are another big, money-making business. In the 1990s, the government released new dietary guidelines urging doctors to advise patients to follow a low-fat diet. It was touted as being good for your heart. You may have assumed this was a positive thing and that a low-fat diet was being promoted as a form of preventative medicine, but unfortunately that wasn't the case. The science was skewed. Processed low-fat foods contain unhealthy hydrogenated fats, usually have a high salt content and sugar is added for flavour (Temple 2018). Around 30 years and countless cases of obesity, diabetes, heart disease and deaths later, the truth has been exposed. I wouldn't recommend you buy anything labelled as low-fat because it will likely have a high sugar content, which is bad for your heart and irritating for your gut (Nguyen et al 2016; La Berge 2008).

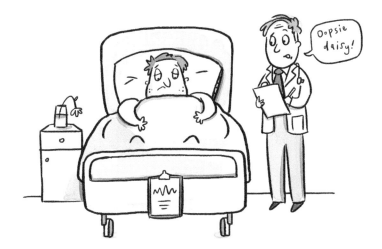

Antidepressants

For many years, some professionals have been questioning the science behind SSRIs because the theory that low serotonin levels are the cause of depression has not given us a complete or satisfactory answer to the problem. I suspect it's a flawed approach because it doesn't take into account a person's unique biochemical imbalances. There may indeed be a correlation between low serotonin and depression in some people, but correlation does not equal causation.

In 2023, the serotonin theory was scientifically disproven in a large umbrella study carried out by Professor Joanna Moncrieff, a professor at University College London, who has worked as a consultant psychiatrist for the NHS for 30 years (Moncrieff et al 2023). I was surprised but pleased when Joanna's study made it into mainstream media because it backed up my belief that we need a brand-new approach to the treatment of mental illness. I can highly recommend Joanna's book, *The Myth of the Chemical Cure* (2007).

Another study of 1,431 people from 38 countries looked into the side effects of SSRIs and concluded that 71 per cent felt emotionally numb, 66 per cent didn't feel like themselves, 66 per cent had sexual difficulties, 40 per cent reported feeling addicted and a whopping 50 per cent reported suicidal feelings as a result of taking antidepressants (Read & Williams 2018). It's scary stuff!

In the long term, SSRIs might actually deplete serotonin (Freeborn 2022). This is because antidepressants block the brain's ability to recycle serotonin. This very quickly depletes reserves, and this is how people become addicted and dependent. Perhaps it also explains why there's a warning on the label, 'for short-term use only'.

Even with very slow, tapered discontinuation, an average of 56 per cent of people experience unpleasant withdrawal effects (Davies & Read 2019). Despite these risks, doctors in England write around 86 million prescriptions a year. These medications are prescribed without any blood tests to check which, if any, neurotransmitters are deficient. Without an accurate diagnosis, doctors can only treat their patients' symptoms and not the root cause.

In psychiatry, every diagnosis is a syndrome. A syndrome is defined as a group of symptoms. But my argument is that a lot of people have a clear biological cause for their mental illness, such as copper overload, a vitamin deficiency or any of the other conditions we've discussed. None of the conditions I've discussed are syndromes. They can all be tested for in a laboratory. This means you know exactly what is causing your brain symptoms and can correct your body chemistry rather than just treating the symptoms with SSRIs. I'm not denying that SSRIs help many people. But there are others who are being failed by symptomatic treatments. I think this approach possibly explains why people on long-term use of SSRIs often experience continuing symptoms and relapses. Think about it. There are no chemical markers for mental illness. Doctors perform blood tests before prescribing drugs like insulin or statins, but not when it comes to psychiatric disorders.

Note to reader: If you're currently taking antidepressants, please don't just stop taking them. There's no disputing that they help millions of people to function and lead a normal life. The people I'm trying to reach with this book are the ones who haven't been helped by the standard medical approach. But if SSRIs work for you, then that's wonderful. If you feel well, that's the most important thing. For the full story, I recommend a couple of wonderful books, *Pharmageddon* (2012) by psychiatrist David Healey and *The Anti-Depressant Fact Book* by Peter R Breggin (2001)..

Interesting titbit

Between 2009 and 2014, the pharmaceutical industry received fines totalling $13 billion for criminal behaviour that included hiding data on the harmful effects of pharmaceutical drugs (Malhotra 2017).

The true stories about low-fat foods and antidepressants demonstrate that scientific research is continually evolving and changing and regularly contradicts itself years down the line. For this reason, I urge you to think outside the box and do your own research. 'Follow the science' has become a popular slogan but perhaps 'Question the science' might be more helpful and progressive.

A true story

I read an article in the *Guardian* (Tickle 2023) about a suicidal 12-year-old girl who was being held in a locked, windowless hospital room for her own safety. She had no personal belongings and her only human contact was through a door hatch. I actually wept reading this article. I wept tears of pain for this little girl and her family, and I wept tears of rage that our medical system is allowed to do this to a vulnerable child. It's totally barbaric and archaic. I mean, what next? Will they be sticking leeches on her and summoning the village priest to perform an exorcism? I wonder if any medical professionals ran tests to search for a biological cause of this child's mental health struggles. It could be something as simple as a vitamin deficiency or copper overload, both of which can cause suicidal feelings but can so easily be corrected with diet and nutritional supplements.

I once heard Patrick Holford say, 'It's better to light a candle than to rage against the darkness.' True stories like this one, my own personal experience of the medical system and the experiences of my clients have caused me to rage against the current medical approach to mental illness. But improving my own health, helping my clients to recover their health and writing this book have been my attempts to light a candle. I pray it leads you out of the darkness.

Chapter 12

Motivation

Motivation is simple – it's just a case of overcoming apathy, if you can be bothered! But on a more serious note, staying motivated and proactive can be tough when you're feeling poorly. It's easy to lose motivation and feel hopeless when facing health challenges, so don't be hard on yourself if you feel apathetic and struggle with motivation.

However, my three-point plan requires you to make dietary and lifestyle changes, and change can be tough – even painful. So, it's important that you master the art of motivation because overcoming health challenges requires a great deal of personal responsibility. And in a society where we're used to handing over the responsibility of our health to a doctor or other healthcare professional, recovery can be challenging.

I recently read an interesting article that said if you wait to feel motivated, you'll wait forever! Instead, you need to choose discipline. I was so struck by the truth in this that I considered changing the title of this chapter to 'Discipline' but I decided it sounded a bit scary!

The tricky bit is getting started. People wait to feel motivated before they take action when in fact it's the action that inspires motivation. So, do something – anything! It doesn't matter how small. It's just important to start moving in the right direction.

The marshmallow test

This was a 1972 Stanford University study into the rewards of delayed gratification (Mischel 2014). A child was given one marshmallow and told they could eat it now, or wait and receive two marshmallows later. The child was then left alone for a short time while being filmed. Some children guzzled down the first marshmallow immediately. Some children sniffed and even licked the marshmallow but didn't eat it. And some of the children waited patiently for the second marshmallow.

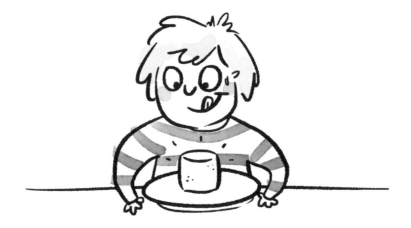

The children from the study were followed up many years later. The results showed that the children who could delay gratification and wait for the second marshmallow were more successful in all areas of their adult lives. So, the moral of this story is, the short-term pain of adapting to my three-point plan is well worth the long-term pleasure of being symptom free, fit and healthy! Eating convenience foods and drinking alcohol may feel great in the short term, but it will only make you feel worse in the long term.

Breaking habits

A habit is a behaviour that has become the norm through constant repetition. It's one of the main factors that governs all human behaviour. So, all we need to do to break a habit is to do things differently, repeat it a few times and hey presto, we've formed a new habit, right? Sounds easy, doesn't it? If only it were that simple! I think it's helpful to tackle change with a positive mindset. So, instead of focusing on breaking your bad habits, I like to reframe them and instead focus on creating new, positive habits. When it comes to our diet and lifestyle, there will be lots of habits that we probably aren't even aware of. Many are subconscious – they've become the norm. Some will be good for us, and some won't.

The point I'm making here is just to be aware that a lot of the foods you eat, the foods you crave and how you eat are just habit, and habits can be changed. Our tastebuds can certainly alter. Remember the first time you tried wine or beer? I'm guessing you didn't love it as much as you do now! Alcohol is usually an acquired taste, and it's the same with many foods. If you consciously replace your morning coffee with herbal tea, red meat with fish or your lunchtime sandwich with a salad, you'll develop new tastes and cravings. Likewise, if you cut out chocolate for a few weeks, you lose the taste for it. Trust me, I've tried!

Sugar is a prime example. Many of my clients who completely cut out sugar say that they lose their craving within two to three weeks. When they finally eat it again, they say it tastes different from how they remember, usually far too sweet. Many processed foods are designed to be addictive so that we will buy them repeatedly. Take a packet of breakfast cereal, for example. Most are chock full of sugars, sweeteners and additives that send pleasure signals to our brain but do little to nourish our bodies. So, it makes me laugh (albeit slightly hysterically) when I see that breakfast cereals are advertised as being fortified with added vitamins, as if it's a good thing! The reason vitamins have to be added is because the cereal grain has been stripped of all its natural nutrients during food processing.

This chapter will assist you in creating new habits around food. Sometimes the tipping point that motivates us to change is when our old habits become more painful to live with than the effort of forming better ones. Changing our eating habits is challenging but living with gut and brain symptoms is undoubtedly much more challenging. I once stuck a very helpful quote on my dressing table mirror: 'You must choose between one of two pains – the pain of discipline or the pain of regret.' It really resonated with me and kept me on the straight and narrow with my diet and lifestyle choices.

Food addiction

I believe that food addiction is on the rise. I'm meeting more and more clients displaying typical food addiction habits: binge eating, obsessive thoughts about food, secret eating, comfort eating, guilty feelings about eating and a complete inability to stick to my three-point plan for more than a week despite desperately wanting to. Sugary foods and processed foods trigger feel-good brain chemicals, like dopamine. Over time these dopamine hits become addictive prompting a negative cycle of craving, overeating and guilt. If you can relate to any of what I'm saying here you may have food addiction, which will make it extremely hard for you to follow my three-point plan. First things first, don't beat yourself up! The food industries are very naughty and they want you addicted! Second, following my three-point plan cuts out all the foods which trigger cravings and this will help quash your addiction. Third, you're probably going to need some help! Recently one of my clients overcame their food addiction with the help of an organisation called Momentum. It's an eight-week programme based on cognitive behavioural therapy and going forward I'll be recommending it to all my clients who feel out of control of their eating.

Pain and pleasure

Two of the greatest motivators are pain and pleasure. Humans will go to great lengths to avoid pain and experience pleasure. Take food as an example. It can be downright painful to deny ourselves our favourite foods, even when we know they're causing our gut and brain symptoms. Take panic attacks as another example. It's natural to want to avoid the pain and trauma of a panic attack, but although avoidance may be the more pleasurable option in the short term, ultimately it leads to pain as your world closes in on you.

What you need to do is attach more pain to a life restricted by gut and brain symptoms and attach massive pleasure to living a healthy, free life. I'm not suggesting this is easy or that the change will happen overnight, but it is possible. A good place to start is to define your motivation. Write down your aims and your reasons for wanting to be well, because to succeed you must have a long-term focus. I recommend you do this in your journal because it's all a part of tracking your progress.

It's important to feel clear about your aims and the results you want to achieve. If you forget the pain and discomfort that motivated you to implement my recommendations in the first place, there's a danger of starting to view your path to wellness as a journey of struggle rather than an uplifting journey to health and happiness. Try not to view my three-point plan as some sort of endurance test! Instead, see the new, empowering approach to your illness as a gift of health that you're giving to yourself.

The second exercise I'd like you to do is to take a moment to think about the characteristics you need to develop to achieve your goals. Write down several traits or values you aspire to and can identify with, such as being strong, tenacious and determined – then write about the times in your life when you experienced those positive feelings. For example, I used to teach in a women's prison, and the first few days of working there were extremely nerve wracking. Yet, when I look back on this experience, I can attach positive feelings of strength and courage to it. I'd like you to do the same and then remind yourself of your positive characteristics daily. These will be values to live your life by.

Another question I'd like you to ask yourself is, do you like yourself enough to make the changes I've recommended? I discussed self-love earlier because it's an important factor in your motivation to heal. If you don't even like yourself, what's the motivation to heal? If this is a problem for you, I recommend you start practising some self-love ASAP. Life is no fun at all if you don't like yourself because wherever you go, you're there! So, stop judging yourself harshly because we all have flaws. You're not on your own. Why not make a list of all your good points? If this sounds too challenging, ask your friends or family to help you with it.

Prep like a boss!

As the lovely fitness expert Joe Wicks says, 'Prep like a boss!' Preparation is everything when making diet and lifestyle changes. If you don't prepare, you may find you simply don't do the things I've recommended. As the saying goes, if you fail to plan, then plan to fail. Make a food shopping list for the week and batch cook meals in advance. Prepare your daily supplements at the start of each day and leave them in a visible place, so you remember to take them.

Arrange to exercise with a friend. Having an exercise buddy is an excellent motivator. Make time for the things that are important to you and book out the time in your diary. Make time to meditate or do food prep in the same way you'd keep a dentist appointment. You should start to feel the benefits very quickly. The improvements in your mental and physical health will be another motivational factor to help you stay focused.

Falling off the wagon

Adapting to the three-point plan is most likely going to be a case of two steps forward and one step back. It's perfectly normal to deviate from time to time, so don't beat yourself up. Learn to anticipate the moods and situations that throw you off track. For example, a stressful day might tempt you to break an alcohol-free resolution and reach for the wine. If you know this to be the case, ensure you have an alternative strategy in place, such as meditating or having a hot bath. Don't allow yourself to make excuses because you need a night off or you deserve a treat. Instead, ask yourself, is this really a treat? Will it ultimately make me feel better or worse?

A somewhat radical but effective method for overcoming the guilt and frustration associated with falling off the wagon is atonement. For example, if you have a day of eating all the wrong foods, you could challenge yourself to a 30-minute run or 100 sit-ups. This method alleviates much of the guilt and helps kick-start motivation again immediately. Setbacks are a normal part of progress, so please don't waste valuable time and energy beating yourself up over your 'fails'. You're only human. Expect failures and learn to deal with them constructively in a proactive manner.

Tell others about your goals

When you share your goals with others, it acts as an accountability measure. People will ask you about them, and that can lead to more motivation. However, be careful about sharing your goals with people who aren't supportive. Take care to surround yourself with like-minded, uplifting souls. Connecting to people who are on the same healing journey as you may also be helpful. It's important to have a support network. If you can share your suffering and your joy, the happier you'll be. Everyone is fighting their own battle. We're all wounded soldiers – but the battle to return to full health, however hard, is always worth it.

As we draw towards the end of the book, I hope you're feeling motivated and inspired to take MASSIVE action! My advice to you is to take one day at a time. If the thought of following my three-point plan feels overwhelming, then break it down. I know you have the discipline to follow my recommendations for one day. So, just take it 24 hours at a time. I have faith in you and I'm praying for you.

Food is medicine

I'm sure you'll have heard the saying, 'It'll either kill or cure you.' I use this saying a lot when explaining to my clients the profound effect our food choices have on our health. Food is medicine, as you'll soon discover when you improve your diet and subsequently feel so much better, both mentally and physically. The aim of my recipes is to remove all the typical gut and brain irritants, ease the workload of your digestive system and create an environment that encourages the proliferation of good gut bacteria. This will allow the gut microbiome to rebalance, regenerate and correct gut dysbiosis.

The following recipes are designed to be as simple as possible. They contain nutritious foods that offer tasty alternatives to the standard Western diet. It can be daunting to adapt to a new way of eating, so I want to make it easy for you. I've been recommending these recipes to my clients for many years now and everyone has found them quick and easy to follow.

Drinks
Aim to drink three litres (five pints) of fluid a day. The drinks I recommend to my clients are filtered water, herbal teas, vegetable juices and bone broth. Please make a commitment to have at least

one freshly squeezed vegetable juice every day. They really help the detoxification process. Another tip to aid detoxification is to add a squeeze of fresh lemon or lime juice to your filtered water. After week one, feel free to choose from my recipes at random. But your first week will look something like this:

Week 1: Rest and repair

I always recommend that my clients spend the first three to seven days 'resting' their gut. The aim of this is to reduce gut and brain inflammation and allow the digestive system to rest and repair. For the first 24 to 72 hours, I recommend that my clients consume only filtered water, herbal teas, vegetable juices, bone broth and bone broth soup. If you are a vegetarian then drinking only filtered water, herbal teas and vegetable juices will still allow your gut to rest but it's the bone broth that heals and repairs. After this initial period, you're likely to be ravenous but try to avoid the temptation to eat excessively and overload your digestive system because it will negate the good work you've just done. Stewed and poached meats are easier to digest and so a slow-cooked stew is an ideal meal for breaking a liquid fast.

Listen to your body, and if you feel you need to stay in the rest and heal phase a bit longer, feel free to stick with soups, bone broth and stew for a week or two. Apologies if this sounds too wishy-washy and unstructured. It's intentional. I want you to get used to listening to your body and eating the foods that feel right for you. There's no such thing as one perfect diet. We're all unique.

After the rest and repair phase, feel free to pick from any of the following recipes at random. Please eat the full range of recommended foods. Remember, the more diverse your diet, the more diverse and happier your gut microbiome will be.

I've included garlic and onion in some of my recipes because they're great for adding flavour but beware these are high-FODMAP foods, which cause wind and bloating in some people, so keep up with your food journal and monitor any reactions. Remember to start your journal for a fortnight before starting the plan.

I've grouped together drinks recipes and then breakfast recipes, lunch recipes, dinner recipes, sweet treats and finally snacks. Cast your eye over the recipes and hopefully this will reassure you that the three-point plan is very doable and is a way of eating you can follow for life. Please feel free to adapt my recipes to suit your needs and tastebuds but ideally don't replace any of my recommended ingredients with sugar, alcohol, dairy, gluten, processed or GM foods.

I don't recommend taking any supplements for the first two weeks, to allow any inflammation in your gut to calm down. Take note of your gut symptoms and when you notice they've improved you can introduce supplements.

Example of a day on the three-point plan

» Upon waking: lie in bed and think of five things to be grateful for.
» Then, weather permitting, sit outside and do 15 minutes of breathing exercises.
» Prep your supplements and food for the day while drinking a mug of bone broth.
» Take a cold shower. If this is too much, take a warm shower and finish off with a 60-second cold blast!
» Make egg muffins for breakfast and take your supplements.
» Have a mid-morning snack such as kale crisps (see 'snacks' below).
» For lunch, have a homemade chicken salad (and take supplements).
» Go for a ten-minute walk and practise mindfulness while walking.
» Have a mid-afternoon snack of berries and coconut yoghurt.
» After work, meet a friend for a yoga class.
» For dinner, have moussaka and vegetables with a tablespoon of ground linseeds sprinkled over the top.
» In the evening, have a freshly squeezed vegetable juice.

» Take your bedtime supplements.
» Lie in bed and follow a ten-minute guided meditation before sleep.

How does that day look to you? It will probably appeal to some readers and for others it will feel overwhelming. If you feel the latter, then I'd advise you to transition slowly. Just incorporate one of my meal suggestions and one of my lifestyle changes for starters and then build up slowly.

Recipe index

Rest and repair: recipes for week one

Fresh mint tea

Pop a handful of fresh mint leaves in a large mug. Pour over boiling water and allow the leaves to steep and the water to cool for a few minutes before drinking.

Lemon and ginger tea

Ginger is anti-inflammatory and great for stimulating the digestion first thing in the morning.

» 1 inch square of fresh root ginger, peeled and sliced.
» Juice of quarter of a lemon.

Pop ingredients in a mug, pour over boiling water, allow to stew for a few minutes and drink.

Vegetable juice

This is my favourite vegetable juice recipe, but feel free to experiment with various vegetable concoctions. You'll probably find in the beginning that you need the sweetness of an apple to make your juices more palatable but try to phase this out as your tastebuds adapt. I recommend buying a masticating juicer as opposed to a centrifugal juicer. This is because a masticating juicer allows higher levels of vitamins and minerals to be extracted. I have an Amzchef cold press masticating juicer.

Ingredients

» Bunch of coriander
» Bunch of celery
» 1 square inch of root ginger
» 1 apple
» Handful of kale

Instructions

Put all the ingredients through a juicer and drink immediately because air exposure makes fruit and veg lose some of their nutritional value.

Bone broth

Bone broth is like a magic elixir! It has a long list of healthful and healing benefits but here are just a few: it's rich in nutrients, heals the gut, soothes the gut, helps overcome food intolerance, reduces inflammation, boosts white blood cells, boosts immunity, protects joints, boosts collagen, improves sleep, supports brain health and increases bone strength (Philpotts 2023). After that long list, you may be asking yourself, 'Is there anything bone broth doesn't do?' Well, the answer is, 'Not much!' I recommend it to all my clients as a first port of call to calm their gut symptoms. The ingredients for this recipe are a tad obscure. See the Resources or speak to your local butcher.

Before the invention of antibiotics, sick patients would be given bone broth because of its wonderful healing and immune-boosting properties. It was a common remedy for influenza back in the day. Our ancestors would have made use of every part of an animal: bones, ligaments, marrow, tendons, skin, feet, and hooves would have been chucked in a pot and simmered slowly over a long period to draw out all their goodness. Animal fats are healing and soothing for the gut. So, I add a teaspoon of organic beef tallow (animal fat) to my mugs of bone broth and recommend my clients do the same. Another option is to add a teaspoon of organic coconut oil, which is antiviral, antifungal and antibacterial and helps fight against pathogens such as *Candida albicans*. I don't recommend shop-bought broth because it's not the real deal. If you want a bone broth that delivers results, you need to make it yourself at home. If the following recipe looks unpalatable and you don't want to drink it neat, then I recommend using bone broth as a stock in your homemade soups. This way, the taste and texture are masked. Consume it daily.

Ingredients

- » Bones (for example, a chicken carcass)
- » Several bone marrows
- » A large handful of chicken feet
- » A splash of apple cider vinegar (look for a label that specifies the vinegar is 'from the mother', which means it contains more beneficial bacteria)
- » 4 sticks of celery
- » 1 onion
- » 2 carrots, diced
- » Several cloves of garlic
- » Filtered water – enough to almost fill the pan or roasting tin

Instructions

Pop all the ingredients into your largest pan or roasting tin so that you can fit in as much water as possible. Pop on a lid and then simmer over a low heat on the hob for a few hours or cook in the oven at 140°C for several hours. The longer you cook it, the more goodness it draws out. Strain the liquid from the ingredients and drink at least one mug a day. It can be frozen.

Bone marrow is full of goodness. After straining off the liquid, throw away all the ingredients except the bone marrow. I eat it immediately while it's still warm. Bone marrow is one of the most healing foods for your gut.

Soups

The base for all your soup recipes should be homemade bone broth. Please avoid shop-bought stock cubes and bouillon powder because they're highly processed. You can invent your own soup and stew recipes. It's really simple. Either on the hob or in a roasting pan in the oven, combine a pint or two of your homemade bone broth along with your favourite combination of meat, vegetables and herbs and cook slowly. You can then blend it into a soup or serve it as it comes, which would be more like a stew. Here are a few recipes to give you some guidance.

Roasted red pepper soup

Serves four.

Ingredients

- » 4 red peppers
- » 2 pints homemade bone broth
- » 2 medium-sized carrots
- » 2 sticks celery
- » 1 large onion, cut into quarters
- » 4 cloves garlic, peeled
- » 1 tin chopped tomatoes
- » Large handful of fresh basil leaves
- » Salt and pepper to taste

Instructions

De-seed the peppers and cut them into quarters. Place on a baking tray with the garlic cloves and onion and lightly brush with melted coconut oil. Cook at 180°C for 25 minutes. Place the bone broth in a pan with the chopped carrots and celery and simmer for ten minutes or until tender. Turn off the heat and add the tin of chopped tomatoes and the basil. Allow to wilt for five minutes before combining all the ingredients and whizzing everything together in a blender.

Tomato soup

Serves four.

Ingredients

- » 1.5 kg tomatoes
- » 1 onion
- » 1 carrot
- » 2 celery sticks
- » Large handful of fresh basil
- » 2 tablespoons coconut oil
- » 2 pints homemade bone broth

Instructions

Halve the tomatoes. Brush with melted coconut oil and roast in the oven at 180°C for 20–25 minutes.

Chop the remaining vegetables and fry gently in coconut oil in a large pan. This should take around ten minutes. When the tomatoes are cooked, add them to the pan along with the basil and bone broth. Simmer gently for ten minutes. Allow to cool slightly before blending.

Celeriac soup

Ingredients

- » 1 small celeriac, peeled and chopped
- » 1 large parsnip, peeled and chopped
- » 4 large handfuls of spinach leaves
- » 1.5 litres of bone broth

Instructions

Combine the ingredients in a pan. Put the lid on and simmer until vegetables are soft. Blend until smooth.

Stew

Serves four.

Stews and casseroles are an excellent meal choice because poaching meat and vegetables makes them easier to digest. I recommend you invest in a slow cooker and experiment with various recipes. Save the juice from this stew and drink it as bone broth.

Ingredients

- » Approx 1 kg of any meat, for example a joint of beef or a whole chicken
- » 3 sticks celery, chopped
- » 1 large onion, chopped
- » 2 carrots, chopped
- » 2 garlic cloves, crushed
- » 1 can of chopped tomatoes

» 1 pint of bone broth

» 1 bouquet garni

Instructions

Put your meat in a casserole dish and almost cover it with water. Pop on a lid and cook slowly for four to six hours on a low heat (140–160°C). One hour before you're ready to eat, add all the vegetables. To make this more of a cottage pie, top the above mixture with celeriac mash. Simply chop, boil and mash half a celeriac and spread it over the stew mixture.

Breakfasts

Breakfast is known as the most important meal of the day, but in my experience, eating first thing in the morning or the last thing at night isn't always advisable for people with gut dysbiosis. The body doesn't digest well while it's asleep, so I recommend being up for at least an hour before eating breakfast. Similarly, I recommend not eating for two or three hours before bed. But, as always, do what feels right for you because we're all unique and different. A great way to stimulate digestion in the morning is with a fresh vegetable juice, a lemon and root ginger tea, or with a tablespoon of apple cider vinegar – or all three!

Homemade kefir

Kefir contains beneficial bacteria that are hugely beneficial to the gut microbiome. I recommend using organic goat's milk.

» 1 pint of goat's milk

» ½ tsp kefir grains

Bring the milk almost to boiling point but not quite. Allow to cool. Put the kefir grains into a clip-top jar and add the milk. Seal the jar and set aside to ferment and thicken for 24 hours. Then strain through a sieve. Storing it in the fridge will slow down the fermentation process slightly. It should keep for seven to ten days. Adding a slice of lemon peel adds a delicious fresh taste.

Linseed porridge

Serves one.

If you add flavoured protein powder, choose carefully to ensure it's dairy, gluten and soya free.

Ingredients

» 50 g golden linseeds, ground
» 10 g sunflower seeds
» 1 scoop vegan protein powder (a variety of flavours are available)

Instructions

Combine ingredients in a pan over a medium heat. Slowly add 50–100 ml of water or almond milk to desired consistency. I sometimes throw in a handful of walnuts or blueberries or raspberries and I always top it with homemade kefir if I have any on the go. If not, I use shop-bought coconut yoghurt.

Egg muffins

It's important to use stable, natural fats when you're cooking because these fats don't change their chemical structure when heated. Lard and coconut oil won't become rancid with heat, so I mostly use them for frying because sunflower oil, olive oil and avocado oil all produce free radicals when heated.

Ingredients

» 6 large eggs
» 2 spring onions, sliced
» 3 slices nitrate-free bacon
» 2 tablespoons fresh chopped parsley
» 2 medium tomatoes, chopped
» 5 mushrooms, chopped
» Asparagus chopped into one-inch pieces

Instructions

Heat the oven to 200°C. Pop bun cases in a muffin tin. Fry the onions, bacon, tomatoes and mushrooms in coconut oil. Whisk the eggs in a separate bowl and then combine all the ingredients. Pour into the muffin tin and top each with the parsley. Bake for 15 minutes or until cooked through.

These keep well in the fridge for three days and make a tasty snack as well as breakfast.

Chia seed pudding

Serves four.

Ingredients

»   40g chia seeds
»   350ml coconut milk or almond milk

Instructions

Combine the ingredients. Mix well. Separate the mixture into four glasses. Refrigerate for four hours or overnight. Serve with a handful of berries.

Fruit salad

Serves one.

Ingredients

»   A small handful of strawberries
»   A small handful of raspberries
»   A small handful of blueberries
»   A sprinkle of chopped nuts
»   A sprinkle of ground linseed

Instructions

Combine all the ingredients. I always add a dollop of coconut yoghurt or homemade kefir.

Scrambled eggs and smoked salmon on almond bread
Serves one.

Ingredients

» 2 slices of almond bread, toasted
» 2 eggs
» 1 smoked salmon slice

Instructions
Melt a teaspoon of coconut oil in a small pan and beat the eggs. Add to the pan and stir continuously until scrambled. With regard to a spread for the toast, use whichever suits you. I use coconut butter, olive oil or ghee.

Lunches
Salads and soups make great lunch options. They're chock full of vitamins and minerals and easy to take to work with you. The variations are endless! You should be continually trying to increase the diversity of good bacteria in your gut and a great way to do this is to add herbs to your salad. I eat a salad on most days. I grow my own herbs and add a different herb every day. Here are a few recipes to give you inspiration.

Almond bread
Ingredients

» 6 eggs, separated
» 1½ cups of ground almonds
» ¼ tsp cream of tartar
» 4 tbsp ghee or lard melted
» ¾ tsp baking powder

Instructions
Whisk egg whites and cream of tartar with an electric hand whisk until light and frothy.

Add all other ingredients and mix well. Pour into a loaf tin and cook for roughly 30 minutes.

You can add any of the following for flavour before cooking: desiccated coconut, onion, olives, herbs, tomatoes.

Grain-free flatbread
Ingredients

- » 250 g almond flour
- » 6 tbsp olive oil
- » 2 tsp sea salt
- » 2 tsp black pepper
- » 1 onion, thinly sliced
- » 3 handfuls finely chopped kale
- » 4 tsp dried or fresh rosemary
- » 225 ml warm water

Instructions

Preheat oven to 200 °C. Combine the almond flour, salt and pepper. Whisk slowly while adding the warm water and three tablespoons of olive oil. Set to one side while you prepare the remaining ingredients. In a frying pan, gently heat the remaining three tablespoons of olive oil and then fry the onions, kale and rosemary for several minutes until softened. Combine with the batter mixture and spread in a deep, greased baking tin. Bake for 15–20 minutes.

Sauerkraut

Makes multiple servings.

Be aware that raw cabbage is low in FODMAPs but fermenting it makes it a high-FODMAP food. Sauerkraut is a mix of vegetables, mainly cabbage, fermented to provide probiotics and other nutrients. I consider it a superfood because of the amount of vitamins, fibre and probiotics it contains. It's easy to make yourself, or you can buy it online. Sauerkraut is a great accompaniment to salads.

Ingredients

- » 1.5 kg pale green or white cabbage
- » 250 g carrot
- » 250 g beetroot
- » 40 g sea salt

Instructions

Shred the veg finely or blitz in a food processor. Pop in a bowl with the salt and massage the salt into the veg for five minutes. Wait ten minutes and then repeat. At this point, you could season with peppercorns or caraway, depending on your personal taste. Put this mixture into an airtight glass jar. Stuff down the mixture so it's covered in its own brine.

Store at room temperature for a minimum of seven days but ideally four weeks. Every few days, open the jar to allow any fermented gases to escape. This part is important because it prevents the jar from exploding. At the same time, taste the mixture. It will become increasingly sour the longer you leave it fermenting. When you decide you like the taste, transfer the mixture to the fridge and consume it regularly. It will keep in the fridge for up to six months.

Bell pepper salad

Serves two.

Ingredients

- » ½ green pepper
- » ½ red pepper
- » ½ yellow pepper
- » A handful of rocket leaves
- » Several basil leaves chopped finely
- » A handful of black olives
- » Grated orange peel to taste (bitter foods aid digestion)

Instructions

De-seed the peppers and cut them into strips. Brush with melted coconut oil and grill. Mix together with the other ingredients.

This can be eaten alone, or you can add protein. I'd recommend a handful of prawns, a cooked salmon fillet, a chicken breast, or a cold, hard-boiled egg.

Mediterranean salad
Ingredients

» Half a romaine lettuce, chopped
» Half an avocado, chopped
» 30 g pitted black olives, chopped
» 3 tomatoes chopped
» Small handful of parsley, chopped
» 1 tbsp extra virgin olive oil
» 1 tbsp fresh lemon juice

Instructions
Combine the ingredients and enjoy alone or add a protein.

Cauliflower rice risotto
Serves two.
This makes a great pack-up.

Ingredients

» 200 g cauliflower, blitzed in a blender
» Tin of tuna in spring water
» Red pepper, de-seeded and sliced
» A handful of parsley, chopped finely
» 2 celery sticks, diced
» 50 g mushrooms, sliced
» 2 sun-dried tomatoes, finely chopped

Instructions
Fry all the vegetables in coconut oil over a medium heat. Last, add the tuna. It can be served hot or cold and if you make extra, it makes a great snack.

Grain-free bacon quiche

Base ingredients

- » 2 cups ground almonds
- » 1 garlic clove crushed
- » 1 tbsp dried oregano
- » 1/3 cup olive oil
- » 3 tbsp water

Filling ingredients

- » 1 garlic clove, crushed
- » 1 onion, sliced
- » Handful of mushrooms, sliced
- » 5 asparagus, chopped
- » 4 rashers nitrate-free bacon, cut into bite-size pieces
- » 6 eggs, beaten

Instructions

Mix the base ingredients and then press into a flan dish. Bake in oven at 180°C for 15 minutes.

Put all other ingredients, apart from the eggs, in a frying pan and fry lightly in coconut oil for ten minutes. Place the fried ingredients in the flan dish. Pour over the eggs and then pop back in the oven for 30–40 minutes.

Mackerel on toast

Serves one.

Ingredients

- » 2 slices of almond bread, toasted
- » 1 tin mackerel in olive oil

Instructions

Drain mackerel and spread over the toast, then pop under a warm grill for three minutes. Serve alone or with a small salad.

Lettuce wrap

Lettuce is a great substitute for traditional wraps such as tortillas.

Ingredients

- » 2 large lettuce leaves
- » 100 g chopped, cooked chicken
- » 5 baby tomatoes, diced
- » 60 g bell pepper, diced
- » Chopped basil, optional
- » 2 tbsp vegan mayonnaise

Instructions

Combine the chicken, tomatoes, bell pepper and basil. Mix with the mayonnaise. Spoon the ingredients onto the lettuce leaves and wrap.

Frittata

Serves two.

Frittata can be eaten cold, so it's ideal for a lunchtime pack-up or a snack.

Ingredients

- » 1 tbsp coconut oil
- » 200 g mushrooms, chopped
- » 100 g asparagus
- » 100 g baby tomatoes, halved
- » 1 tablespoon chopped basil
- » 1 tsp mixed herbs
- » 5 eggs, beaten

If you'd like a vegetarian frittata then the above ingredients make a tasty dish. Alternatively, you could add a tin of tuna or anchovies, or a handful of prawns.

Instructions

Heat the coconut oil in a pan. Add the mushrooms and asparagus. Cook on a high heat for several minutes, stirring regularly. Turn down the heat and add garlic and baby tomatoes. Cook for a further couple of minutes before adding the eggs and the rest of the ingredients. Cook on a low heat until the eggs are cooked through.

Fermented fish

Fermented foods are healing and healthful for the gut.

Ingredients

» 2 wild-caught salmon steaks, boneless and skinless, cut into chunks
» 2 small white onions, peeled and sliced
» 2 tsp peppercorns
» 1 tbsp fresh coriander, chopped
» 2 tbsp sea salt
» 2 tbsp manuka honey
» 3 bay leaves
» 1 tsp dill
» 5 tbsp whey from your homemade kefir

Instructions

Place all the ingredients in a large mason jar. Top up each jar with filtered water. Seal jar with a lid. Allow to ferment at room temperature for a week. Once opened, store in fridge. Goes well with salad.

Jacket sweet potato
Ingredients

» 1 sweet potato
» Filling of your choice. Tuna mixed with vegan mayonnaise is my personal fave.

Instructions

Bake the potato in the oven or microwave. Add the filling and serve with a salad or sauerkraut.

Dinners

Salmon steak

Serves one.

Ingredients

- » 1 salmon steak
- » 2 handfuls of watercress
- » 1 carrot, grated
- » ¼ of a bulb of fennel, cut into thin strips (fennel aids peristalsis and calms the gut)

Instructions

Sit the salmon on a piece of greaseproof paper, drizzle over half the lemon juice, fold the foil over to make a pouch. Put in the oven at 180°C for 20 minutes. Arrange the other ingredients on a plate. Sit the salmon on top and serve.

Roasted vegetables

Serves one.

Ingredients

- » Half an aubergine, sliced thickly
- » 7 baby tomatoes, whole
- » 10 sun-dried tomatoes, chopped
- » 1 sweet red pepper, sliced thickly
- » 5 Brussels sprouts
- » Half a courgette, sliced thickly
- » A handful of nuts and a handful of seeds

Instructions

Put the ingredients on a baking tray, season with salt, pepper and dried mixed herbs. Drizzle with melted coconut oil and mix well. Cover with foil and bake for approximately 25–35 minutes at 180°C, stirring once.

Courgette noodles

Courgette noodles make a great substitute for pasta and rice. If you don't have a spiraliser you can use a vegetable peeler to slice the courgette into ribbons.

Ingredients

- » 1 large courgette, sliced into ribbons
- » 1 tbsp coconut oil
- » 1 tsp sea salt
- » Handful of chopped basil
- » Handful of pine nuts

Instructions

Heat the coconut oil in a frying pan. Add the pine nuts and toast until golden brown. They easily burn so keep a close eye on them. Add the courgette ribbons to the pan and cook for several minutes until softened. Add the basil for a minute to warm through and then serve immediately. This dish makes a great accompaniment to a chicken breast.

Vegetable kebabs

Ingredients

- » 4 tablespoons manuka honey
- » 3 tsp grainy mustard
- » 4 tbsp olive oil
- » 1 courgette, thickly sliced
- » 2 red bell peppers, cut into one-inch pieces
- » 1 small aubergine, cut into chunks

- » 2 handfuls of small mushrooms
- » 10 baby tomatoes
- » 1 tsp dried oregano
- » Black pepper and salt to taste

If using wooden skewers, soak them in water for 30 minutes to stop them burning. Heat the oven to 180°C. Combine the honey, mustard, oil, oregano, salt and pepper in a large bowl. Add the vegetables and mix well to coat with the honey mixture. Thread the vegetables onto the skewers. Cook for 20–30 minutes.

Bolognese
Serves two.

Ingredients

- » 500 g beef mince
- » 5 rashers of nitrate-free bacon, chopped
- » 1 onion, chopped
- » 3 garlic cloves, crushed
- » 3 celery stalks, chopped
- » A sprinkling of dried rosemary
- » For the bolognese sauce:
- » 1 can of chopped tomatoes
- » 1 large handful of basil leaves, finely chopped
- » 3 tbsp tomato puree
- » 100 ml bone broth

Instructions
Fry the bacon, onion, garlic, celery and rosemary on a low heat for five minutes, stirring regularly. Increase the heat and add the beef. Stir continually for several minutes. Reduce the heat and add the bolognese sauce ingredients. Cover and simmer for an hour. Serve with courgette noodles.

Vegetable curry

You can't beat a curry! It's tasty, versatile and easy to make. Here in York, we're blessed with a wonderful shop that sells you the exact mix of spices needed for various curries. Curry making has never been easier. All you do is chop up 1 kg of your chosen ingredients, add the little pack of spices and cook. The good news is that these little curry packs are available to buy online at spicebox.co.uk Alternatively, you can make your own curry from scratch.

Ingredients

- » 50 g coconut butter
- » 250 g mushrooms
- » 100 g green beans
- » 1 carrot, diced
- » 1 red pepper, sliced
- » Handful of cashews
- » 1 onion
- » 4 garlic cloves
- » 6 tbsp olive oil
- » 1 tsp fennel seeds
- » 1 tsp cumin seeds
- » 1 tbsp grated ginger
- » ½ tsp ground turmeric
- » 1 tsp curry powder
- » 400 g tin chopped tomatoes

Instructions

Melt the coconut butter in a large pan then cook all the vegetables on high for five minutes, stirring continuously. Add the tin of tomatoes and all the other ingredients and cook on low for 20 minutes or until the vegetables are softened. If you like your curry mild, stir in a few tbsp of coconut yoghurt before serving. Garnish with a handful of coriander.

Moussaka

Serves four.

Ingredients

- » 3 tbsp olive oil
- » 2 large aubergines, sliced
- » 500 g minced lamb
- » 4 large tomatoes, sliced
- » 1 tin chopped tomatoes
- » 2 tsp dried rosemary
- » 2 tbsp tomato puree

For the topping:

- » 2 eggs
- » 300 g coconut yoghurt
- » 50 g vegan cheese, grated

Instructions

Toss the aubergine slices in olive oil, lay on baking trays and bake in the oven for 20 minutes at 180°C. Fry the lamb mince and rosemary for five minutes. Add the tin of chopped tomatoes and the tomato puree. Cook on a low heat for a further five minutes. Next, you're going to layer the ingredients in a casserole dish: a layer of the mince mixture, then a layer of sliced tomatoes, then the aubergine. Keep repeating until all the ingredients are in the casserole dish. Then whisk together the eggs and coconut and pour over the top. Finally, sprinkle over the grated cheese. Pop in the oven at 170°C for 40 minutes.

Stir fry

Make double the amount, and you have a pack-up for lunch the following day.

Ingredients

- » 2 carrots, diced
- » 1 courgette, thinly sliced
- » 1 carrot, thinly sliced
- » 100 g mushrooms
- » 100 g green beans, top and tailed and cut in half
- » 1 red bell pepper, thinly sliced
- » 2 tbsp fresh root ginger, thinly slice
- » Handful of water chestnuts
- » 150 g protein-rich food such as chicken, prawns, tuna
- » 2 tsp Chinese five spice

Instructions

Heat some olive oil in a wok or large frying pan. Add the chicken breast (or other protein) and Chinese five spice and stir until the chicken (or other protein) is sealed. Add the vegetables and cook through.

Tuna steak and ratatouille

Serves two.

Ingredients

- » 2 tuna steaks, preferably wild caught
- » 1 heaped tbsp coconut oil
- » 1 small onion, chopped
- » 1 clove garlic, crushed
- » 1 small aubergine, sliced
- » 1 large courgette, sliced
- » 1 red bell pepper, sliced
- » 3 tomatoes, sliced

» 1 tin chopped tomatoes, drained
» A handful of basil, chopped

Instructions

Individually wrap the tuna steaks in foil with a teaspoon of coconut oil. Bake at 180°C for 20 minutes. Put the remaining coconut oil in a frying pan. Add the onion, aubergine, courgette, bell pepper and fry on a high heat for five minutes, stirring continually. Lower the heat and add the garlic and tomatoes. Fry for a further five minutes before adding the tinned tomatoes and basil. Stir well and serve with the tuna steak.

Puddings

Lime bombs

Serves two.

Ingredients

» 6 tbsp coconut butter
» 6 tbsp coconut oil
» 5 tbsp shredded coconut
» 3 tbsp lime juice
» 2 tbsp lime zest

Instructions

Whizz together the ingredients in a food processor. Store the mixture in a freezer for 30 minutes until it firms up. Take out and separate the mixture into ten balls. Roll each ball in shredded coconut to coat.

Coconut treats

Ingredients

» 200 g flaked coconut
» 100 g coconut butter

» 100 g coconut oil
» 200 g raspberries or strawberries

Instructions

Set aside the coconut flakes. Combine the other ingredients in a food processor and blend thoroughly. Form into little balls and roll in the coconut flakes.

Fruity sundae
Ingredients

» 200 g coconut yoghurt
» 50 g raspberries
» 75 g sliced strawberries
» 25 g coconut flakes
» 2 tbsp pumpkin seeds

Instructions

Fry the coconut flakes and pumpkin seeds for a few minutes until they're gently toasted. In small glasses, layer up the ingredients in any order you like. They'll keep in the refrigerator for three days.

Nutty chocolate
Ingredients

» 2 tbsp chopped nuts
» 90 g bar of dark chocolate, 75 per cent cocoa
» 1 heaped tbsp of peanut butter

Instructions

Combine the ingredients in a glass bowl and heat gently over boiling water. Mix thoroughly and then spoon the mixture into an ice-cube tray and pop in the freezer to set.

Ice cream

Serves four.

OK, this isn't really ice cream – but it's a tasty substitute!

Ingredients

» 1 tin of coconut milk
» 1 punnet of berries

Instructions

Mix together and pop in the freezer.

Snacks

I know I've mentioned a few shop-bought, processed foods here, but they make a tasty occasional treat.

» Crudités make a delicious, healthy snack. Try celery, carrot, cucumber, raw cauliflower or any other veg of your choice and dip into hummus or guacamole.
» Low-sugar fruits such as berries.
» Roasted sweet potato wedges or roasted celeriac wedges.
» Cold, hard-boiled eggs.
» Celery and pate or celery and almond butter.
» Grain-free flatbread dipped in olive tapenade.
» Olives with seaweed thins.
» Apple and nut butter.
» Dark chocolate. My personal favourite is Hu organic chocolate bars. Available in a variety of flavours.
» Kale crisps. Toss a few handfuls of kale in olive oil. Sprinkle over a teaspoon of sea salt and a teaspoon of dried rosemary. Pop in the oven at 180°C for ten minutes. Stir halfway through cooking. Keeps for a day.
» Toasted coconut flakes.

Conclusion

'Before you heal someone, ask if he's willing to give up the things that made him sick.' – attributed to Hippocrates

The great news is that following my three-point plan is relatively simple. All it takes is a little bit of effort. You obviously already have the motivation to feel well or you wouldn't be reading this book. Listen to your body: some foods will make you feel sluggish, and some will make you feel energetic. After eating, take note of how you feel and avoid those foods that make you feel lethargic in the future. Your body really does know best! Your food journal will help you with this. Always read ingredient labels and know exactly what you're eating.

Every action has a reaction, so every thought you think and every food you eat is affecting your future health and wellbeing. You'll get out of my three-point plan what you put in. The more you nurture and care for yourself, the better you'll feel. The discipline to stick to my three-point plan will come naturally when you see how much better you feel. The improvement in your gut and brain symptoms should keep you on the straight and narrow. Don't look at the three-point plan as some sort of endurance test! Instead, reframe it and look at it as a time to feast on nutrient-dense foods and nurture yourself. Eat fresh, whole foods in their natural state, keep yourself rested and calm and your body will do the rest. Get back to a simple, clean-living way of life wherever you can.

A note of caution

If you've thoroughly explored everything I suggest in this book and feel no better, I suggest you enlist the support of a professional who can suggest some different blood tests. And take heart: if you believe your mental health problems are not psychosomatic, then you're probably right. After all, no one knows you better than you. But sometimes it can be tricky to detect the biological cause of your problems. Take the story of the woman in an earlier chapter who was allergic to the pesticide sprays surrounding her home. Who would have believed that pesticide sprays were causing her deep depression? She was fortunate to discover the source of her troubles. You may never be 100 per cent free of your gut and brain symptoms but I've seen lots of people feel life-changingly better. Read all the books I recommend and keep expanding your knowledge. Hopefully something will lead you to the cause of your gut and brain symptoms.

Some of my clients make a marvellous recovery despite never discovering the exact cause of their brain symptoms. These are the patients who can't afford to pay privately for the blood tests I recommend. But my three-point plan brings the workings of the body back into harmony for the majority of people who consult me. You have nothing to lose by giving it your best shot. I know for sure that your body will appreciate it. So, trust the process. Good luck and God bless.

References and resources

Articles and research papers cited

Achufusi, T G O, Sharma, A et al (2020) 'Small intestinal bacterial overgrowth: Comprehensive review of diagnosis, prevention, and treatment methods'. *Cureus* 12(6).

Aizawa, E, Tsuji, H et al (2016) 'Possible association of Bifidobacterium and Lactobacillus in the gut microbiota of patients with major depressive disorder'. *Journal of Affective Disorders* 202.

Akpinar, S & Karadag, M G (2022) 'Is vitamin D important in anxiety or depression? What is the truth?'. *Nutrition and the Brain* 11.

Almahayni, O & Hammond, L (2024) 'Does the Wim Hof Method have a beneficial impact on physiological and psychological outcomes in healthy and non-healthy participants? A systematic review'. *PloS One* 19(3).

Almatroodi, S A, Alsahli, M A et al (2022) 'Berberine: An important emphasis on its anticancer effects through modulation of various cell signaling pathways'. *Molecules* 27(18).

Alt, K W, Al-Ahmad, A & Woelber, J P (2022) 'Nutrition and health in human evolution – past to present'. *Nutrients* 14(17).

Anand, P, Kunnumakkara, A B et al (2008) 'Cancer is a preventable disease that requires major lifestyle changes'. *Pharmaceutical Research* 25(9).

Anglin, R E, Samaan, Z et al (2013) ' Vitamin D deficiency and depression in adults: Systematic review and meta-analysis'. *The British Journal of Psychiatry* 202.

Appleton, J (2018) 'The gut–brain axis: Influence of microbiota on mood and mental health'. *Integrative Medicine* 17(4).

Arasaradnam, R P, Brown, S et al (2018) 'Guidelines for the investigation of chronic diarrhoea in adults'. *Gut* 67.

Ariel, H & Cooke, J P (2019) 'Cardiovascular risk of proton pump inhibitors'. *Methodist DeBakey Cardiovascular Journal* 15(3).

Arnarson, A (2023) '7 signs and symptoms of magnesium deficiency'. Healthline. URL: healthline.com/nutrition/magnesium-deficiency-symptoms

Bai, N (2024) 'Pilot study shows ketogenic diet improves severe mental illness'. Stanford Medicine, URL: med.stanford.edu/news/all-news/2024/04/keto-diet-mental-illness.html

Baranwal, N, Yu, P K & Siegel, N S (2023) 'Sleep physiology, pathophysiology, and sleep hygiene. *Progress in Cardiovascular Diseases* 77.

Basmaciyan, L, Bon, F et al (2019) '*Candida albicans* interactions with the host: Crossing the intestinal epithelial barrier'. *Tissue Barriers* 7(2).

BBC News (2002) 'Doctors want GM crop ban'. URL: news.bbc.co.uk/1/hi/scotland/2494267.stm

Berry, J (2023) 'Everything you need to know about berberine'. MedicalNewsToday. URL: medicalnewstoday.com/articles/325798

Blacher, S (2023) 'Emotional Freedom Technique (EFT): Tap to relieve stress and burnout'. *Journal of Interprofessional Education & Practice* 30.

Block, G, Jensen, C D et al (2007) 'Usage patterns, health, and nutritional status of long-term multiple dietary supplement users: A cross-sectional study'. *Nutrition Journal* 6.

Boyle, N B, Lawton, C & Dye, L (2017) 'The effects of magnesium supplementation on subjective anxiety and stress – a systematic review'. *Nutrients* 9(5).

Bradley, J (2023) 'Antibiotics are a staple of modern medicine and save millions of lives every year. But they can be harming the normal bacterial system our health relies on'. BBC Future. URL: bbc.com/

future/article/20230825-do-antibiotics-really-wipe-out-your-gut-bacteria

Bradley, P (2019) 'Refined carbohydrates, phenotypic plasticity and the obesity epidemic'. *Medical Hypotheses* 131.

Brauer-Nikonow, A & Zimmermann, M (2022) 'How the gut microbiota helps keep us vitaminized'. *Cell Host & Microbe* 30(8).

Brazier, Y (2024) 'What is a food intolerance?'. MedicalNewsToday. URL: medicalnewstoday.com/articles/263965

Bremner, J D (2006) 'Traumatic stress: Effects on the brain'. *Dialogues in Clinical Neuroscience* 8(4).

Brown, M J (2023) '8 health benefits of probiotics'. Healthline. URL: healthline.com/nutrition/8-health-benefits-of-probiotics

Brownley, K A, Von Holle, A et al (2013) 'A double-blind, randomized pilot trial of chromium picolinate for binge eating disorder: Results of the Binge Eating and Chromium (BEACh) study'. *Journal of Psychosomatic Research* 75(1).

Bueno-Notivol, J, Gracia-García, P et al (2021) 'Prevalence of depression during the COVID-19 outbreak: A meta-analysis of community-based studies'. *International Journal of Clinical and Health Psychology* 21(1).

Busby, E, Bold, J et al (2018) 'Mood disorders and gluten: It's not all in your mind! A systematic review with meta-analysis'. *Nutrients* 10(11).

Bush, B & Welsh, H (2015) 'Hidden hunger: America's growing malnutrition epidemic'. *Guardian* 10 Feb 2015. URL: theguardian.com/lifeandstyle/2015/feb/10/nutrition-hunger-food-children-vitamins-us

Campbell-McBride, N (2004) *Gut and Psychology Syndrome*. Medinform Publishing.

Cao, B, Sun X-Y et al (2018) 'Association between B vitamins and schizophrenia: A population-based case-control study'. *Psychiatry Research* 259.

Carolbetty (2009) 'Redheads, inflammation and celiac disease'. URL: blessedwithred.blogspot.com/2009/12/redheads-inflammation-and-celiac.html

Carter, S (2019) 'Origins of orthomolecular medicine. *Integrative Medicine (Encinitas)* 18(3).

Chandler, J (2021) 'Menopause around the world'. Mindset Health. URL: mindsethealth.com/matter/menopause-around-the-world

Chen, J, Song, W & Zhang, W (2023) 'The emerging role of copper in depression'. *Frontiers in Neuroscience* 17.

Cherney K (2023) 'What to know about pyrrole disorder'. Healthline. URL: healthline.com/health/pyrrole-disorder

Chong, R Q, Gelissen, I et al (2021) 'Do medicines commonly used by older adults impact their nutrient status?'. *Exploratory Research in Clinical and Social Pharmacy* 3.

Chugani, H T, Behen M E et al (2001) 'Local brain functional activity following early deprivation: A study of postinstitutionalized Romanian orphans'. *Neuroimage* 14(6).

Cresci, G A & Bawden, E (2015) 'Gut microbiome: What we do and don't know'. *Nutrition in Clinical Practice* 30(6).

Crews, M G, Taper, L J & Ritchey, S J (1980) 'Effects of oral contraceptive agents on copper and zinc balance in young women'. *American Journal of Clinical Nutrition* 33(9).

Cui, X, McGrath J J et al (2021) 'Vitamin D and schizophrenia: 20 years on'. *Molecular Psychiatry* 26(7).

Cullinan, M & Newey, S (2024) 'Groundup chicken waste fed to cattle may be behind bird flu outbreak in US cows'. *Telegraph* 9 April 2024.

Davidson, J R, Abraham, K et al (2003) 'Effectiveness of chromium in atypical depression: A placebo-controlled trial'. *Biological Psychiatry* 53(3).

Davies, J, & Read, J (2019) 'A systematic review into the incidence, severity and duration of antidepressant withdrawal effects: Are guidelines evidence-based?'. *Addictive Behaviors* 97.

Deruelle, F & Baron, B (2008) 'Vitamin C: Is supplementation necessary for optimal health?'. *Journal of Alternative and Complementary Medicine* 14(10).

Deville, L (2022) 'Methylation defects'. URL: drlaurendeville.com/methylation-defects

Dillon, S (2018) 'We learn nothing about nutrition, claim medical students'. BBC News. URL: bbc.co.uk/news/health-43504125

Dohan, F C (1966) 'Wheat "consumption" and hospital admissions for schizophrenia during World War II: A preliminary report'. *American Journal of Clinical Nutrition* 18(1).

Dona, A, Arvanitoyannis, I S (2009) 'Health risks of genetically modified foods'. *Critical Reviews in Food Science and Nutrition* 49(2).

Dos Santos, R D, Viana, M L et al (2010) 'Glutamine supplementation decreases intestinal permeability and preserves gut mucosa integrity in an experimental mouse model'. *Journal of Parenteral and Enteral Nutrition* 34(4).

Drago, S, El Asmar, R et al (2006) 'Zonulin and gut permeability: Effects on celiac and non-celiac intestinal mucosa and intestinal cell lines'. *Scandinavian Journal of Gastroenterology* 41(4).

El-Tawil, A M (2016) 'Colorectal cancers and chlorinated water'. *World Journal of Gastrointestinal Oncology* 8(4).

Ensari, A (2014) 'The malabsorption syndrome and its causes and consequences'. *Pathobiology of Human Disease* 2014.

Ernst, E (2000) 'Herbal medicines: Where is the evidence?'. *BMJ (Clinical research ed.)* 321(7258).

Fond, G, Macgregor, A et al (2013) 'Fasting in mood disorders: Neurobiology and effectiveness. A review of the literature'. *Psychiatry Research* 209(3).

Food for the Brain (n.d.) 'The shrinking brain: Are we dumbing down?'. URL: foodforthebrain.org/the-shrinking-brain-are-we-dumbing-down

Food for the Brain Foundation (2024) 'The impact of food intolerances on mental health'. URL: foodforthebrain.org/the-impact-of-food-intolerances-on-mental-health

Fraczek, B, Pieta, A et al (2021) 'Paleolithic diet – effect on the health status and performance of athletes?'. *Nutrients* 13(3).

Freeborn, J (2022) 'Low serotonin might not cause depression, but why do SSRIs still work?' MedicalNewsToday. URL: medicalnewstoday.com/articles/low-serotonin-might-not-cause-depression-but-why-do-ssris-still-work

Freese, J, Klement, R J et al (2017) 'The sedentary revolution: Have we lost our metabolic flexibility?'. *F1000 Research* 6.

Fujimori, S (2015) 'What are the effects of proton pump inhibitors on the small intestine?' *World Journal of Gastroenterology* 21(22).

Gardner, A & Boles, R G (2011) 'Beyond the serotonin hypothesis:

Mitochondria, inflammation and neurodegeneration in major depression and affective spectrum disorders'. *Progress in Neuro-Psychopharmacology and Biological Psychiatry* 35(3).

Gasperi, V, Sibilano, M et al (2019) 'Niacin in the central nervous system: An update of biological aspects and clinical applications'. *International Journal of Molecular Sciences* 20(4).

GBD 2017 Diet Collaborators (2019) 'Health effects of dietary risks in 195 countries, 1990–2017: A systematic analysis for the Global Burden of Disease Study 2017'. *Lancet* 393(10184).

Gerretsen, I (2024) 'Why power naps might be good for our health'. BBC Future. URL: bbc.com/future/article/20240126-why-power-naps-might-be-good-for-our-health

Ghimpeteanu, O M, Pogurschi, E N et al (2022) 'Antibiotic use in livestock and residues in food a public health threat: A review'. *Foods* 11(10).

Godfrey, P S, Toone, B K et al (1990) 'Enhancement of recovery from psychiatric illness by methylfolate'. *Lancet* 336(8712).

Gonsalkorale, W M, Miller, V et al (2003) 'Long term benefits of hypnotherapy for irritable bowel syndrome'. *Gut* 52(11).

Gøtzsche, P C (2014) 'Our prescription drugs kill us in large numbers'. *Polskie Archiwum Medycyny Wewnetrznej* 124(11).

Greenblatt, J (2021) 'Zinc: An essential but overlooked element in the fight against anorexia'. Psychiatry Redefined. URL: psychiatryredefined.org/zinc-an-essential-element-in-the-fight-against-anorexia

Grønli, O, Kvamme, J M et al (2013) 'Zinc deficiency is common in several psychiatric disorders'. *PloS One* 8(12).

Grosso, G, Galvano, F et al (2014) 'Omega-3 fatty acids and depression: Scientific evidence and biological mechanisms'. *Oxidative Medicine and Cellular Longevity* 2014.

Grosso, G, Pajak, A, et al (2014) 'Role of omega-3 fatty acids in the treatment of depressive disorders: A comprehensive meta-analysis of randomized clinical trials'. *PloS One* 9(5).

Gunnars, K (2023) 'How to optimize your omega-6 to omega-3 ration'. Healthline. URL: healthline.com/nutrition/optimize-omega-6-omega-3-ratio

Gunston, J (2023) 'Novak Djokovic's life and career-changing gluten-free diet'. Olympics.com. URL: olympics.com/en/news/novak-djokovic-gluten-free-diet

Gurib-Fakim, A (2006) 'Medicinal plants: Traditions of yesterday and drugs of tomorrow'. *Molecular Aspects of Medicine* 27(1).

Han, Y, Wang, B et al (2022) 'Vagus nerve and underlying impact on the gut microbiota–brain axis in behavior and neuro-degenerative diseases'. *Journal of Inflammation Research* 15.

Harvard Health Publishing (2019) 'Stress and the sensitive gut'. URL: health.harvard.edu/newsletter_article/stress-and-the-sensitive-gut

Heber, D & Carpenter, C L (2011) 'Addictive genes and the relationship to obesity and inflammation'. *Molecular Neurobiology* 44(2).

Herdiana, Y (2023) 'Functional food in relation to gastroesophageal reflux disease (GERD)'. *Nutrients* 15(16).

Hodges, R E & Minich, D M (2015) 'Modulation of metabolic detoxification pathways using foods and food-derived components: A scientific review with clinical application'. *Journal of Nutrition and Metabolism* 2015.

Hoffer, A (1970) 'Pellagra and schizophrenia'. *Psychosomatics* 11(5).

Hoffer, L J (2008) 'Vitamin therapy in schizophrenia'. *Israel Journal of Psychiatry and Related Sciences* 45(1).

Hosea, L & Salvidge, R (2023) '"Forever chemicals" found in drinking water sources across England'. *Guardian* 28 November 2023.

Howren, M B, Lamkin, D M et al (2009) 'Associations of depression with C-reactive protein, IL-1, and IL-6: A meta-analysis'. *Psychosomatic Medicine* 71(2).

Hrncir, T (2022) 'Gut microbiota dysbiosis: Triggers, consequences, diagnostic and therapeutic options'. *Microorganisms* 10(3).

Hrncirova, L, Machova, V et al (2019) 'Food preservatives induce proteobacteria dysbiosis in human – microbiota associated Nod2-deficient mice'. *Microorganisms* 7(10).

Hsu, H H, Leung, W H & Hu, G C (2016) 'Treatment of irritable bowel syndrome with a novel colonic irrigation system: A pilot study'. *Techniques in Coloproctology* 20(8).

Humphrey, L, Fu, R et al (2008) 'Homocysteine level and coronary heart disease incidence: A systematic review and meta-analysis'. *Mayo Clinic Proceedings* 83(11).

Hunter, D J (2005) 'Gene–environment interactions in human diseases'. *Nature Reviews Genetics* 6.

Hwang, W J, Lee, T Y et al (2020) 'The role of estrogen receptors and their signalling across psychiatric disorders'. *International Journal of Molecular Science* 22(1).

Ianiro, G, Pecere, S et al (2016) 'Digestive enzyme supplementation in gastrointestinal diseases'. *Current Drug Metabolism* 17(2).

iPhysio (2014) 'Scientists link drinking milk with osteoporosis'. URL: iphysio.io/osteoporosis

Jackson, E, Shoemaker, R et al (2017) 'Adipose tissue as a site of toxin accumulation'. *Comprehensive Physiology* 7(4).

Jalili, M, Vahedi, H et al (2019) 'Effects of vitamin D supplementation in patients with irritable bowel syndrome: A randomized, double-blind, placebo-controlled clinical trial'. *International Journal of Preventive Medicine* 10.

Jamar, G, Ribeiro, D A & Pisani, L P (2020) 'High-fat or high-sugar diets as trigger inflammation in the microbiota–gut–brain axis'. *Critical Reviews in Food Science and Nutrition* 61(5).

Jamil, A, Gutlapalli, S et al (2023) 'Meditation and its mental and physical health benefits in 2023'. *Cureus* 15(6).

Johnson, K (2016) 'Before steroids, Russians secretly studied herbs'. National Geographic. URL: nationalgeographic.com/culture/article/long-before-doping-scandals--russians-were-studying-performance

Johnston, R, Poti, J M & Popkin, B M (2014) 'Eating and aging: Trends in dietary intake among older Americans from 1977–2010'. *The Journal of Nutrition, Health & Aging* 18(3).

Kawoos, Y, Wani, Z A et al (2017) 'Psychiatric co-morbidity in patients with irritable bowel syndrome at a tertiary care center in Northern India'. *Journal of Neurogastroenterology and Motility* 23(4).

Kennedy, D O (2016) 'B vitamins and the brain: Mechanisms, dose and efficacy – a review'. *Nutrients* 8(2).

Khalili, H, Huang, E et al (2012) 'Use of proton pump inhibitors and risk of hip fracture in relation to dietary and lifestyle factors: A prospective cohort study'. *BMJ* 344.

Kines, K & Krupczak, T (2016) 'Nutritional interventions for gastroesophageal reflux, irritable bowel syndrome, and hypochlorhydria: A case report'. *Integrative Medicine (Encinitas)* 15(4).

Kleinridders, A, Cai, W et al (2015) 'Insulin resistance in brain alters dopamine turnover and causes behavioral disorders'. *Proceedings of the National Academy of Sciences of the United States of America* 112(11).

Kober, M M & Bowe, W P (2015) 'The effect of probiotics on immune regulation, acne, and photoaging'. *International Journal of Women's Dermatology* 1(2).

Kordestani-Moghadam, P, Assari, S et al (2020) 'Cognitive impairments and associated structural brain changes in metabolic syndrome and implications of neurocognitive intervention'. *Journal of Obesity and Metabolic Syndrome* 29(3).

Kossewska, J, Bierlit, K & Trajkovski, V (2022) 'Personality, anxiety, and stress in patients with small intestine bacterial overgrowth syndrome. The Polish Preliminary Study'. *International Journal of Environmental Research and Public Health* 20(1).

Kubala, J (2022) 'Zinc: Everything you need to know'. Healthline. URL: healthline.com/nutrition/zinc

La Berge, A F (2008) 'How the ideology of low fat conquered America'. *Journal of the History of Medicine and Allied Sciences* 63(2).

Lane, M M, Gamage, E et al (2022). 'Ultra-processed food consumption and mental health: A systematic review and meta-analysis of observational studies'. *Nutrients* 14(13).

Lee, C, Lau, E et al (2019) 'Protective effects of vitamin D against injury in intestinal epithelium'. *Pediatric Surgery International* 35(12).

Lee, D Y W, Li, Q Y et al (2021) 'Traditional Chinese herbal medicine at the forefront battle against COVID-19: Clinical experience and scientific basis'. *Phytomedicine* 80.

Lee, K H, Cha, M et al (2020) 'Neuroprotective effects of antioxidants in the brain'. *International Journal of Molecular Science* 21(19).

Levinta, A, Mukovozov, I & Tsoutsoulas C (2018) 'Use of a gluten-free diet in schizophrenia: A systematic review'. *Advances in Nutrition* 9(6).

Levy, J (2018) '10 antinutrients to get out of your diet... and life'. Dr Axe. URL: draxe.com/nutrition/antinutrients

Levy, J (2023) 'Hydrochloric acid: Stomach acid that defends against GERD, Candida & leaky gut'. Dr Axe. URL: draxe.com/nutrition/hydrochloric-acid

Levy, J (2024) 'Aflatoxin: How to avoid this common food carcinogen'. URL: draxe.com/nutrition/aflatoxin

Linhart, C, Talasz, H et al (2017) 'Use of underarm cosmetic products in relation to risk of breast cancer: A case-control study'. *eBioMedicine* 6 June 2017.

Lovell, R (n.d.) 'How modern food can regain its nutrients'. BBC Future. URL: bbc.com/future/bespoke/follow-the-food/why-modern-food-lost-its-nutrients

Lyon, L (2018) '"All disease begins in the gut": Was Hippocrates right?'. *Brain* 141(3).

Maes, M, Kubera, M & Leunis, J C (2008) 'The gut–brain barrier in major depression: Intestinal mucosal dysfunction with an increased translocation of LPS from gram negative enterobacteria (leaky gut) plays a role in the inflammatory pathophysiology of depression'. *Neuro Endocrinology Letters* 29(1).

Magan, N, Aldred, D et al (2010) 'Limiting mycotoxins in stored wheat'. *Food Additives & Contaminants: Part A* 27(5).

Mahindru, A, Patil, P et al (2023) 'Role of physical activity on mental health and wellbeing: A review. *Cureus* 15(1).

Makharia, A, Catassi, C & Makharia, G K (2015) 'The overlap between irritable bowel syndrome and non-celiac gluten sensitivity: A clinical dilemma'. *Nutrients* 7(12).

Makunts, T, Alpatty, S et al (2019) 'Proton-pump inhibitor use is associated with a broad spectrum of neurological adverse events including impaired hearing, vision, and memory'. *Scientific Reports* 9(1).

Malhotra, A (2017) 'Finance trumps patients at every level – UK healthcare needs an enquiry'. *Guardian* 21 Nov 2017. URL: theguardian.com/healthcare-network/2017/nov/21/finance-trumps-patients-uk-healthcare-needs-inquiry

Manheimer, E, Cheng, K et al (2012) 'Acupuncture for treatment of irritable bowel syndrome'. *The Cochrane Database of Systematic Reviews* 2012(5).

Mathias, M (2018) 'Autointoxication and historical precursors of the microbiome–gut–brain axis'. *Microbial Ecology in Health and Disease* 29(2).

Mattson, M P, Moehl, K et al (2018) 'Intermittent metabolic switching, neuroplasticity and brain health'. *Nature Reviews Neuroscience* 19.

Mayer E A (2011) 'Gut feelings: The emerging biology of gut–brain communication'. *Nature Reviews Neuroscience* 12(8).

McCulloch, M (2023) '9 signs and symptoms of vitamin B6 deficiency'. Healthline. URL: healthline.com/nutrition/vitamin-b6-deficiency-symptoms

MHRA (2020) 'Isotretinoin: Reminder of important risks and precautions'. Medicines and Healthcare products Regulatory Agency. URL: gov.uk/drug-safety-update/isotretinoin-roaccutane-reminder-of-important-risks-and-precautions

Michaëlsson, G, Ahs, S et al (2003) 'Gluten-free diet in psoriasis patients with antibodies to gliadin results in decreased expression of tissue transglutaminase and fewer Ki67+ cells in the dermis'. *Acta Dermato-Venereologica* 83(6).

Miller, A H, Haroon, E et al (2013) 'Cytokine targets in the brain: Impact on neurotransmitters and neurocircuits'. *Depression and Anxiety* 30(4).

Miller, C L & Dulay, J R (2008) 'The high-affinity niacin receptor HM74A is decreased in the anterior cingulate cortex of individuals with schizophrenia'. *Brain Research Bulletin* 77(1).

Molberg, O, Uhlen, A K et al (2005) 'Mapping of gluten T-cell epitopes in the bread wheat ancestors: Implications for celiac disease'. *Gastroenterology* 128(2).

Moncrieff, J, Cooper, R E et al (2023) 'The serotonin theory of depression: A systemic umbrella review of the evidence'. *Molecular Psychiatry* 28.

Müller-Lissner, S, Kaatz, V et al (2005) 'The perceived effect of various foods and beverages on stool consistency'. *European Journal of Gastroenterology & Hepatology* 17(1).

Munro H N (1977) 'How well recommended are the recommended dietary allowances?'. *Journal of the American Dietetic Association* 71(5).

Mustafe, H N (2021) 'Morphohistometric analysis of the effects of Coriandrum sativum on cortical and cerebellar neurotoxicity'. *Avicenna Journal of Phytomedicine* 11(6).

Nanayakkara, W S, Skidmore, P M L et al (2016) 'Efficacy of the low FODMAP diet for treating irritable bowel syndrome: The evidence to date'. *Clinical and Experimental Gastroenterology* 9.

National Cancer Institute (n.d.) 'Mistletoe extracts (PDQ) – health professional version'. URL: cancer.gov/about-cancer/treatment/cam/hp/mistletoe-pdq

National Library of Medicine (2003) 'Overview of food fortification in the United States and Canada'. URL: ncbi.nlm.nih.gov/books/NBK208880

Nguyen, P K, Lin, S & Heidenreich, P (2016) 'A systematic comparison of sugar content in low-fat vs regular versions of food'. *Nutrition & Diabetes* 6(1).

NHS (2021) 'Peppermint oil'. URL: nhs.uk/medicines/peppermint-oil

NIH (2013) 'Common genetic factors found in 5 mental disorders'. National Institutes of Health. URL: nih.gov/news-events/nih-research-matters/common-genetic-factors-found-5-mental-disorders

Och, A, Och, M et al (2022) 'Berberine, a herbal metabolite in the metabolic syndrome: The risk factors, course, and consequences of the disease'. *Molecules* 27(4).

Otten, A T, Bourgonje, A R et al (2021) 'Vitamin C supplementation in healthy individuals leads to shifts of bacterial populations in the gut-a pilot study'. *Antioxidants* 10(8).

Paone, P, Cani, P D (2020) 'Mucus barrier, mucins and gut microbiota: The expected slimy partners?'. *Gut* 69.

Parliament (2017) *The Long-term Sustainability of the NHS and Adult Social Care Contents*. Chapter 6. URL: publications.parliament.uk/pa/ld201617/ldselect/ldnhssus/151/15109.htm

Patterson, E, Wall, R et al (2012) 'Health implications of high dietary omega-6 polyunsaturated fatty acids'. *Journal of Nutrition and Metabolism* 5 April 2012.

Peckham, S & Awofeso, N (2014) 'Water fluoridation: A critical review of the physiological effects of ingested fluoride as a public health intervention'. *Scientific World Journal* 26 Feb 2014.

Peckham, S, Lowery, D & Spencer, S (2015) 'Are fluoride levels in drinking water associated with hypothyroidism prevalence in England? A large observational study of GP practice data and fluoride levels in drinking water'. *Journal of Epidemiology Community Health* 69(7).

Pei, D, Hsieh, C H et al (2006) 'The influence of chromium chloride-containing milk to glycemic control of patients with type 2 diabetes mellitus: A randomized, double-blind, placebo-controlled trial'. *Metabolism: Clinical and Experimental* 55(7).

Penckofer, S, Quinn, L et al (2012) 'Does glycemic variability impact mood and quality of life?'. *Diabetes Technology & Therapeutics* 14(4).

Pendyala, S, Walker, J M et al (2012) 'A high-fat diet is associated with endotoxemia that originates from the gut'. *Gastroenterology* 142(5).

Perez-Cornago, A (2020) 'Commentary: Dairy milk intake and breast cancer risk: Does an association exist, and what might be the culprit?'. *International Journal of Epidemiology* 49(5).

Periyasamy, S, John, S et al (2019) 'Association of schizophrenia risk with disordered niacin metabolism in an Indian genome-wide association study'. *JAMA Psychiatry* 76(10).

Perry, B D (2002) 'Childhood experience and the expression of genetic potential: What childhood neglect tells us about nature and nurture'. *Brain and Mind* 3(1). URL: researchgate.net/publication/225759011_Childhood_Experience_and_the_Expression_of_Genetic_Potential_What_Childhood_Neglect_Tells_Us_About_Nature_and_Nurture

Philpotts, R (2023) 'Top 5 health benefits of bone broth'. BBC Good Food. URL: bbcgoodfood.com/howto/guide/health-benefits-of-bone-broth

Qiao, C, Lauver, D A et al (2013) 'Atorvastatin-induced cardiac function impairment'. *FASEB Journal* 27(S1).

Queensland Brain Institute (2023) 'Half of world's population will experience a mental health disorder'. Harvard Medical School. URL: hms.harvard.edu/news/half-worlds-population-will-experience-mental-health-disorder

Rafiei, R, Ataie, M et al (2014) 'A new acupuncture method for management of irritable bowel syndrome: A randomized double blind clinical trial'. *Journal of Research in Medical Sciences* 19(10).

Rappaport, J (2017) 'Changes in dietary iodine explains increasing incidence of breast cancer with distant involvement in young women'. *Journal of Cancer* 8(2).

Ravindran, J, Agrawal, M et al (2011) 'Alterations of blood–brain barrier permeability by T-2 toxin: Role of MMP-9 and inflammatory cytokines'. *Toxicology* 280(1–2).

Read, J, & Williams, J (2018) 'Adverse effects of antidepressants reported by a large international cohort: Emotional blunting, suicidality, and withdrawal effects'. *Current Drug Safety* 13(3).

Redzic S, Hashmi M F, Gupta V (2023) 'Niacin deficiency'. URL: ncbi. nlm.nih.gov/books/NBK557728

Rigoni, C (2020) 'Pyrrole disorder (pyroluria) – everything you need to know'. URL: drcarrierigoni.com.au/blog/pyrroles-disorder

Rippere, V (1984) 'Some varieties of food intolerance in psychiatric patients: An overview'. *Nutrition and Health* 3(3).

Roman Viñas, B, Ribas Barba, L et al (2011) 'Projected prevalence of inadequate nutrient intakes in Europe'. *Annals of Nutrition & Metabolism* 59(2–4).

Sahu, P, Thippeswamy, H & Chaturvedi, S K (2022) 'Neuropsychiatric manifestations in vitamin B12 deficiency'. *Vitamins and Hormones* 119.

Salim, S (2014) 'Oxidative stress and psychological disorders'. *Current Neuropharmacology* 12(2).

Sambu, S, Hemaram, U et al (2022) 'Toxicological and teratogenic effect of various food additives: An updated review'. *BioMed Research International* 2022.

Sangle, P, Sandhu, O et al (2020) 'Vitamin B12 supplementation: Preventing onset and improving prognosis of depression'. *Cureus* 12(10).

Sankowski, R, Mader, S et al (2015) 'Systemic inflammation and the brain: Novel roles of genetic, molecular, and environmental cues as drivers of neurodegeneration'. *Frontiers in Cellular Neuroscience* 9.

Sapone, A, Bai, J C et al (2012) 'Spectrum of gluten-related disorders: Consensus on new nomenclature and classification'. *BMC Medicine* 10.

Sarkar, A, Lehto, S M et al (2016) 'Psychobiotics and the manipulation of bacteria–gut–brain signals'. *Trends in Neurosciences* 39(11).

Sarris, J, Logan A C et al (2015) 'Nutritional medicine as mainstream in psychiatry'. *Lancet Psychiatry* 2(3).

Sasso, J M, Ammar, R M et al (2023) 'Gut microbiome–brain alliance: A landscape view into mental and gastrointestinal health disorders'. *ACS Chemical Neuroscience* 14(10).

Scherf, K A (2019) 'Immunoreactive cereal proteins in wheat allergy, non-celiac gluten/wheat sensitivity (NCGS) and celiac disease'. *Current Opinion in Food Science* 25.

Schiffman, S S (2023) 'Toxicological and pharmacokinetic properties of sucralose-6-acetate and its parent sucralose: *in vitro* screening assays'. *Journal of Toxicology and Environmental Health*, Part B 26(6).

Seidell, J C (2000) 'Obesity, insulin resistance and diabetes – a worldwide epidemic'. *The British Journal of Nutrition* 83 Suppl 1.

Sethi, S & Ford, J M (2022) 'The role of ketogenic metabolic therapy on the brain in serious mental illness: a review'. *Journal of Psychiatry and Brain Science* 7(5).

Severance, E, Gressitt, K et al (2016) 'Candida albicans exposures, sex specificity and cognitive deficits in schizophrenia and bipolar disorder'. *npj Schizophrenia* 2.

Shafiei, Z, Esfandiari, F et al (2020) 'Parasitic infections in irritable bowel syndrome patients: Evidence to propose a possible link, based on a case–control study in the south of Iran'. *BMC Research Notes* 13.

Shah, T Z, Ali, A B et al (2013) 'Effect of nicotinic acid (vitamin B3 or niacin) on the lipid profile of diabetic and non-diabetic rats'. *Pakistan Journal of Medical Sciences* 29(5).

Sharma, L L, Teret, S P & Brownell, K D (2010) 'The food industry and self-regulation: Standards to promote success and to avoid public health failures'. *American Journal of Public Health* 100(2).

Sherman, L (2023) 'Oxidative stress: Your FAQs answered'. Healthline. URL: healthline.com/health/oxidative-stress-your-faqs-answered

Shipowick, C D, Moore, C B et al (2009) 'Vitamin D and depressive symptoms in women during the winter: A pilot study'. *Applied Nursing Research* 22(3).

Silva, E C, Wadt, et al (2017) 'Natural variation of selenium in Brazil nuts and soils from the Amazon region'. *Chemosphere* 188.

Singh, S, Sharma, P et al (2022) 'Impact of environmental pollutants on gut microbiome and mental health via the gut–brain axis'. *Microorganisms* 10(7).

Smith, A D & Refsum, H (2021) 'Homocysteine – from disease marker to disease prevention'. *Journal of Internal Medicine* 290(4).

Smith, A P (2016) 'Chewing gum and stress reduction'. *Journal of Clinical and Translational Research* 2(2).

Son, H, Baek, J H et al (2018) 'Glutamine has antidepressive effects through increments of glutamate and glutamine levels and glutamatergic activity in the medial prefrontal cortex'. *Neuropharmacology* 143.

Spagnuolo, R, Cosco, C et al (2017) 'Beta-glucan, inositol and digestive enzymes improve quality of life of patients with inflammatory bowel disease and irritable bowel syndrome'. *European Review for Medical and Pharmacological Sciences* 21(2 Suppl).

Spreadbury, I (2012) 'Comparison with ancestral diets suggests dense acellular carbohydrates promote an inflammatory microbiota, and may be the primary dietary cause of leptin resistance and obesity'. *Diabetes, Metabolic Syndrome and Obesity* 5.

Stone, W (2024) 'Patients say keto helps with their mental illness. Science is racing to understand why'. NPR. URL: npr.org/sections/health-shots/2024/01/27/1227062470/keto-ketogenic-diet-mental-illness-bipolar-depression

Studo, N, Chida, Y et al (2004) 'Postnatal microbial colonization programs the hypothalamic-pituitary-adrenal system for stress response in mice'. *Journal of Physiology* 558(1).

Sukalingam, K, Ganesan, K et al (2015) 'An insight into the harmful effects of soy protein: A review'. *La Clinica Terapeutica* 166(3).

Sun, J, Wang, F et al (2016) 'Antidepressant-like effects of sodium butyrate and its possible mechanisms of action in mice exposed to chronic unpredictable mild stress'. *Neuroscience Letters* 618.

Tardy, A E, Pouteau, E et al (2020) 'Vitamins and minerals for energy, fatigue and cognition: A narrative review of the biochemical and clinical evidence'. *Nutrients* 12(1).

Temple, N J (2018) 'Fat, sugar, whole grains and heart disease: 50 years of confusion'. *Nutrients* 10(1).

Thomas, D (2007) 'The mineral depletion of foods available to us as a nation (1940–2002) – a review of the 6th edition of McCance and Widdowson'. *Nutrition and health* 19(1–2).

Tickle, L (2023) 'Mother of suicidal girl held in locked hospital room "frightened" for child's life'. Guardian 7 Feb 2023. URL: theguardian. com/society/2023/feb/07/mother-of-suicidal-girl-held-in-locked-hospital-room-frightened-for-childs-life

Tiwari, A & Balasundaram, P (2023) 'Public health considerations regarding obesity'. *StatPearls* [*Internet*]. URL: ncbi.nlm.nih.gov/ books/NBK572122

Toriizuka, K, Mizowaki, M & Hanawa, T (2000) 'Menopause and anxiety: Focus on steroidal hormones and GABAA receptor'. *Nihon Yakurigaku Zasshi* 115(1).

Totten, M S, Davenport, T S et al (2023) 'Trace minerals and anxiety: A review of zinc, copper, iron, and selenium'. *Dietetics* 2(1).

Twardowska, A, Makaro, A et al (2022) 'Preventing bacterial translocation in patients with leaky gut syndrome: Nutrition and pharmacological treatment options'. *International Journal of Molecular Science* 23(6).

Ulas, A S, Cakir, A & Erbas, O (2022) 'Gluten and casein: Their roles in psychiatric disorders'. *Journal of Experimental and Basic Medical Sciences* 3(1).

Van De Walle, G (2023) '5 science-based benefits of 5-HTP (plus dosage and side effects)'. Healthline. URL: healthline.com/nutrition/5-htp-benefits

Van der Vossen, E W J, Davids, M et al (2023) 'Gut microbiome transitions across generations in different ethnicities in an urban setting: The HELIUS study'. *Microbiome* 11(1).

Veeresham, C (2012) 'Natural products derived from plants as a source of drugs'. *Journal of Advanced Pharmaceutical Technology & Research* 3(4).

Venturelli, S, Leischner, C et al (2021) 'Vitamins as possible cancer biomarkers: Significance and limitations'. *Nutrients* 13(11).

Walsh, W J, Glab, L B et al (2004) 'Reduced violent behaviour following biochemical therapy'. *Physiology & Behavior* 82(5).

Watson, K (2019) 'Zinc deficiency'. Healthline. URL: healthline.com/health/zinc-deficiency

Watson, K (2023) 'What is lazy bowel syndrome?'. Healthline. URL: healthline.com/health/lazy-bowel

WebMD (2023) 'What to know about vitamins and mental health'. URL: webmd.com/vitamins-and-supplements/what-to-know-about-vitamins-and-mental-health

Weinhold, B (2006) 'Epigenetics: The science of change'. *Environmental Health Perspectives* 114(3).

Wilson, J L (2014) 'Clinical perspective on stress, cortisol and adrenal fatigue'. *Advances in Integrative Medicine* 1(2).

Winstone, J K, Pathak, K V et al (2022) 'Glyphosate infiltrates the brain and increases pro-inflammatory cytokine TNFa: Implications for neurodegenerative disorders'. *Journal of Neuroinflammation* 19(1).

Woodford, K B (2021) 'Casomorphins and gliadorphins have diverse systemic effects spanning gut, brain and internal organs'. *International Journal of Environmental Research and Public Health* 18(15).

WorldHealth.net (2020) 'NHS doctors looking to change the system to be more preventive'. URL: worldhealth.net/news/nhs-doctors-looking-change-system-be-more-preventive

Xiang, M, Zheng, L et al (2022) 'Intestinal microbes in patients with schizophrenia undergoing short-term treatment: Core species identification based on co-occurrence networks and regression analysis'. *Frontiers in Microbiology* 13.

Xie, Y, Liu, X & Zhou, P (2020) 'In vitro antifungal effects of berberine against Candida spp. in planktonic and biofilm conditions'. *Drug Design, Development and Therapy* 14.

Yang, Y, Ke, Y et al (2024) 'Navigating the B vitamins: Dietary adversity, microbial synthesis, and human health'. *Cell Host & Microbe* 32(1).

Ye, Y, Liu, X et al (2021) 'Efficacy and safety of berberine alone for several metabolic disorders: A systematic review and meta-analysis of randomized clinical trials'. *Frontiers in Pharmacology* 12.

Yee, B E, Richards, P et al (2020) 'Serum zinc levels and efficacy of zinc treatment in acne vulgaris: A systematic review and meta-analysis'. *Dermatologic Therapy* 33(6).

Young, L M, Pipingas, A et al (2019) 'A systematic review and meta-analysis of B vitamin supplementation on depressive symptoms, anxiety, and stress: Effects on healthy and "at-risk" individuals'. *Nutrients* 11(9).

Zhan, Y, Han, J et al (2021) 'Berberine suppresses mice depression behaviors and promotes hippocampal neurons growth through regulating the miR-34b-5p/miR-470-5p/BDNF axis'. *Neuropsychiatric Disease and Treatment* 17.

Zhou, L, Chen, L et al (2019) 'Food allergy induces alteration in brain inflammatory status and cognitive impairments'. *Behavioural Brain Research* 364.

Zhou, Q, Verne, M L et al (2019) 'Randomised placebo-controlled trial of dietary glutamine supplements for postinfectious irritable bowel syndrome'. *Gut* 68(6).

Further reading

Axe, J (2019) *Keto Diet: Your 30-day plan to lose weight, balance hormones, boost brain health, and reverse disease*. Orion Spring.

Blythman, J (2015) *Swallow this: Serving up the food Industry's darkest secrets*. Fourth Estate.

Braly, J & Holford, P (2003) *The H Factor: The fast new way to dramatically improve your health and add 20 years to your life*. Piatkus.

Braly, J & Holford, P (2003) *The H Factor Solution: Depression and Schizophrenia*. Basic Health Publications.

Breggin, P R (2001) *The Anti-Depressant Fact Book*. Da Capo Lifelong Books.

Campbell, T C (2005) *The China Study*. BenBella Books.

Clarke, H (1995) *The Cure for All Diseases*. New Century Press.

Cohen, A (2015) *A Course in Miracles Made Easy: Mastering the journey from fear to love*. Hay House UK.

Crawford, M & Marsh, D E (2023) *The Shrinking Brain*. Filament Publishing.

Gundry, S R (2017) *The Plant Paradox: The hidden dangers in 'healthy' foods that cause disease and weight gain*. Harper.

Hari, J (2019) *Lost Connections: Why you're depressed and how to find hope.* Bloomsbury Publishing.

Healey, D (2012) *Pharmageddon.* University of California Press.

Hof, W (2020) *The Wim Hof Method.* Rider.

Holford, P (2004) *The Optimum Nutrition Bible.* Piatkus.
   Holford, P (2010) *Stress and Fatigue: The drug-free guide to de-stressing and raising your energy levels.* Piatkus.

Holford, P (2017) *Improve Your Digestion: How to make your gut work for you and not against you.* Piatkus.

Holford, P & McDonald Joyce, F (2011) *The 9 Day Liver Detox: The definitive detox diet that delivers results.* Piatkus.

Malhotra, A & O'Neill, D (2017). *The Pioppi Diet: The 21-day anti-diabetes lifestyle plan.* Penguin.

Manson, M (2016) *The Subtle Art of Not Giving A F*ck: A counterintuitive approach to living a good life.* Harper.

McLelland, J (2018) *How to Starve Cancer.* Agenor Publishing.

Mischel, W (2014) *The Marshmallow Test: Mastering self-control.* Little, Brown & Co.

Moncrieff, J (2007) *The Myth of the Chemical Cure.* Palgrave Macmillan.

Myhill, S & Robinson, C (2018) *The Infection Game: Life is an arms race.* Hammersmith Health Books.

Overeaters Anonymous (2018) *The Twelve Steps and Twelve Traditions of Overeaters Anonymous.* Overeaters Anonymous.

Palmer, C M (2022) *Brain Energy.* BenBella Books.

Pelz, M (2015) *The Reset Factor.* CreateSpace.

Pelz, M (2022) *Fast Like a Girl.* Hay House.

Perlmutter, D (2013) *Grain Brain: The surprising truth about wheat, carbs, and sugar – your brain's silent killers.* Yellow Kite.

Proctor, B (2021) *Change Your Paradigm, Change Your Life.* G&D Media.

Puri, B & Boyd, H (2005) *The Natural Way to Beat Depression.* Hodder.

Tolle, E (2001) *The Power of Now: A guide to spiritual enlightenment.* Yellow Kite.

Trickett, S (2009) *Coping Successfully with Panic Attacks.* Sheldon Press.

Truss, C O (1985) *The Missing Diagnosis.* Missing Diagnosis.

Van Tulleken, C (2023) *Ultra-Processed People.* Cornerstone Press.

Vorderman, C, Chohan, K & Bean, A (2001) *Carol Vorderman's Detox for Life: The 28 day detox diet and beyond*. Virgin Books.

Walsh, W J (2012) *Nutrient Power*. Skyhorse Publishing.

White, E (2014) *Erica White's Beat Candida Cookbook: Over 340 recipes with a 4-point plan for attacking candidiasis*. Thorsons.

Wilson, J L (2001) *Adrenal Fatigue: The 21st century stress syndrome*. Smart Publications.

Wilson, W G (1952) *Twelve Steps and Twelve Traditions*. Alcoholics Anonymous.

Young, R & Redford Young, S (2010) *The pH Miracle: Balance your diet, reclaim your health*. Balance.

Other useful links

Meditations

Headspace is an app that has guided meditations, mindfulness and sleep guides. URL: headspace.com/meditation

Food and snacks

Green Pastures Farm: for organic, pasture-raised meat and the ingredients needed for bone broth. URL: greenpasturesfarm.co.uk

Suma Coop: for whole foods, paraben-free body care products and environmentally-friendly (and human-friendly) cleaning products. URL: suma.coop

Qualified nutritionists

Find one in your area via associationfornutrition.org or bant.org.uk

Private doctors

Natural Health Worldwide: a website created by Dr Sarah Myhill, who aims to empower patients and encourages a natural approach to health. You can order tests and find recommended doctors and healthcare professionals through this site. URL: naturalhealthworldwide.com

Dr Miriam Mikicki: mikickimedical.com

Complementary therapies

The Research Council for Complementary Medicine lists all the various professional bodies for different therapies. Follow the links to find qualified practitioners in your area. URL: rccm. org.uk

Tests

Food allergy testing at York Test: yorktest.com, 01904 410410.

Hair mineral analysis: hairanalysisuk.com

Blood tests without a doctor's request: bloodtest.co.uk

Food for the Brain Foundation: Homocysteine and HbA1C (glucose control) testing and much more. This is an awesome charity. Please check out the website and get involved. URL: foodforthebrain.org

Smart Nutrition: Offers blood tests and follow-up consultations with nutritionists. URL: smartnutrition.co.uk

Newson Health: Treatment and support for women during the menopause and perimenopause. URL: newsonhealth.co.uk

Individual WellBeing Diagnostic Laboratories: privatehealth.co.uk/ clinics/1094-individual-wellbeing-diagnostic-laboratories

Recommended supplement suppliers

- » biocare.co.uk
- » bobbyshealthyshop.co.uk
- » british-supplements.net
- » highernature.com
- » holfordirect.com
- » lambertshealthcare.co.uk
- » nutriadvanced.co.uk
- » salesatdrmyhill.co.uk
- » solgar.co.uk
- » viridian-nutrition.com

Other websites of interest

Professor Campbell-McBride's website details all of her wonderful work into gut and psychology syndrome: gapsdiet.com

Walsh Research Institute: Better health through biochemistry. URL: www.walshinstitute.org

Institute for Optimum Nutrition (ION): www.ion.ac.uk

Bristol Stool Chart: england.nhs.uk/wp-content/uploads/2023/07/Bristol-stool-chart-for-carer-web-version.pdf

The Natural Choice, supplier of herbs recommended by Dr Hulda Clarke: the-natural-choice.co.uk

Understanding colon/bowel cancer: cancerresearchuk.org/about-cancer/bowel-cancer

Brad Yates – Tap with Brad. URL: youtube.com/channel/UCiHZMZejDS4RIxDdBwoie9A

Beat Eating Disorders (Momentum). URL: beateatingdisorders.org.uk/get-information-and-support/get-help-for-myself/momentum

About the author

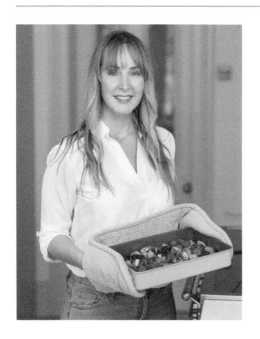

Joanne Mordue qualified as a nutritional therapist in 2010. Over the years, she inadvertently ended up specialising in irritable bowel syndrome because it's so prevalent. As her clients' digestive health improved, she found their mental health symptoms often improved too. This led to Joanne's personal interest in the gut–brain connection. As a result, she formulated a three-point plan comprising dietary changes, lifestyle changes and nutritional supplements as a holistic approach to her clients' health and wellbeing. Joanne lives and works in York in the north of England.